SANITATION AND HYGIENE IN EAST ASIA

WHO Library Cataloguing in Publication Data

Sanitation and hygiene in East Asia.

1. Sanitation. 2. Hygiene. 3. Far East. 4. Asia, Southeastern.

ISBN 978 92 9061 483 8   (NLM Classification: WA 670)

© World Health Organization 2010

All rights reserved. Publications of the World Health Organization can be obtained from WHO Press, World Health Organization, 20 Avenue Appia, 1211 Geneva 27, Switzerland (tel.: +41 22 791 3264; fax: +41 22 791 4857; e-mail: bookorders@who.int). Requests for permission to reproduce or translate WHO publications – whether for sale or for noncommercial distribution – should be addressed to WHO Press, at the above address (fax: +41 22 791 4806; e-mail: permissions@who.int). For WHO Western Pacific Regional Publications, request for permission to reproduce should be addressed to the Publications Office, World Health Organization, Regional Office for the Western Pacific, P.O. Box 2932, 1000, Manila, Philippines, Fax. No. (632) 521-1036, email: publications@wpro.who.int

The designations employed and the presentation of the material in this publication do not imply the expression of any opinion whatsoever on the part of the World Health Organization concerning the legal status of any country, territory, city or area or of its authorities, or concerning the delimitation of its frontiers or boundaries. Dotted lines on maps represent approximate border lines for which there may not yet be full agreement.

The mention of specific companies or of certain manufacturers' products does not imply that they are endorsed or recommended by the World Health Organization in preference to others of a similar nature that are not mentioned. Errors and omissions excepted, the names of proprietary products are distinguished by initial capital letters.

All reasonable precautions have been taken by the World Health Organization to verify the information contained in this publication. However, the published material is being distributed without warranty of any kind, either expressed or implied. The responsibility for the interpretation and use of the material lies with the reader. In no event shall the World Health Organization be liable for damages arising from its use.

Table of contents

Acknowledgements vi
Preface vii
Executive summary viii
Introduction 1
Demography and health 3
Status of sanitation 8
Achieving the sanitation targets 14
Monitoring sanitation 17
Why is hygiene so important? 22
Investing in sanitation and hygiene 24
Stakeholders participation 27
Sanitation and hygiene in schools and health care facilities 31
How are institutions organized to face the sanitation challenge? 34
Why is this all happening? 38
Intercountry and interregional interaction 43
Way forward 45
Bibliographic references 51
Acronyms 53
Annex 1   Declaration of the First East Asia Ministerial Conference
             on Sanitation and Hygiene 55
Annex II   Charter of the Regional Forum on Environment
             and Health – Framework for Cooperation 58
Annex III   Sanitation coverage in East Asia in 1990 and 2008 according
             to the JMP statistics review of 2010 65

Figures

Figure 1	Urban and rural population of East Asia, 1990, 2008 and 2015 (projected)	3
Figure 2	Distribution of causes of death among children under 5 years old in East Asian countries	4
Figure 3	Under-five mortality rate per 1000 live births in East Asian countries, 1990 and 2007	5
Figure 4	"Waves" of human contamination from human excreta, animal excreta and animal products	6
Figure 5	Annual incidence rates of diarrhoeal diseases per 1000 population in the East Asian countries, 2004	7
Figure 6	Deaths due to diarrhoeal diseases per 100 000 population in the East Asian countries in 2004	7
Figure 7	Proportion of the East Asia population using an improved, shared or other unimproved sanitation facility or practising open defecation, 1990, 2008	10
Figure 8	Proportion of the population in East Asian countries using an improved, shared or other unimproved sanitation facility or practising open defecation, 2008	10
Figure 9	Population in East Asia using an improved, shared or other unimproved sanitation facility or practising open defecation, 1990, 2008	11
Figure 10	Urban and rural proportions of people with access to improved sanitation in East Asian countries, 2008	12
Figure 11	Urban and rural populations without access to improved sanitation in East Asia, 2008	13
Figure 12	Proportion of people using improved sanitation in 2008, projected proportion of people using improved sanitation in 2015 and respective country MDG sanitation target in East Asian countries	14
Figure 13	Change in the proportion of people with improved sanitation between 1990 and 2008 and projection of change in East Asia between 2008 and 2015	15
Figure 14	Change in population with improved and unimproved sanitation between 1990 and 2008 and projection of change between 2008 and 2015 in East Asia	16
Figure 15	Proportion of people using improved urban sanitation in East Asian countries, according to official national statistics and the JMP, 2008	17
Figure 16	Proportion of people using improved rural sanitation in East Asian countries, according to official national statistics and the JMP, 2008	18
Figure 17	Perception of the effectiveness of hygiene education programmes in selected East Asian countries	22
Figure 18	Percentage of public schools having adequate sanitation facilities in selected East Asian countries	31
Figure 19	Proportion of public hospitals and health care centres with adequate sanitation facilities in selected East Asian Countries	32
Figure 20	Governmental responsibility for sanitation in East Asian countries	34

Figure 21   Level of training and sufficiency of sanitation personnel in East Asia 36
Figure 22   Proportion of population in East Asia without access to improved
             sanitation facilities, 1990, 2008 42

Tables

Table 1   Groups of sanitation categories 8
Table 2   Types of sanitation facilities considered hygienically adequate
          or inadequate by East Asian countries 19
Table 3   Initiatives, plans or programmes on sanitation as reported by East Asian countries 26
Table 4   Recommendations for the improvement of sanitation and hygiene
          in public schools and health establishments in East Asian countries 33
Table 5   Recommendations and issues on the sanitation and hygiene institutional
          framework in East Asian countries 35
Table 6   Recommendations for sanitation and hygiene human resources improvement
          in East Asian countries 37
Table 7   Constraints for sanitation improvement as perceived by East Asian countries 38
Table 8   Top constraints for sanitation improvement as perceived by East Asian countries 39
Table 9   How to enhance cooperation and exchange of information
          among East Asian countries 44

Boxes

Box 1   WHO and UNICEF Joint Monitoring Programme for Water Supply
         and Sanitation (JMP) 9
Box 2   National water supply and sanitation sector assessments 20
Box 3   Economic impact of sanitation in South-East Asia 25
Box 4   A Cambodian village decides to bring sanitation closer to home 29
Box 5   Why people want latrines 29
Box 6   Approaches to improve sanitation 40
Box 7   The resilience of sanitation systems to climate change 40
Box 8   Use of treated excreta and urine in agriculture 41
Box 9   The International Year of Sanitation 43
Box 10   Things to do in East Asia 47

Acknowledgements

This report was prepared by the Thematic Working Group on Water, Hygiene and Sanitation for the Second East Asia Ministerial Conference on Sanitation and Hygiene, Manila, Philippines, 27 – 29 January 2010.

A number of dedicated professionals in the sanitation sector contributed valuably to the preparation of this report. The Chairman of the Thematic Working Group on Water, Hygiene and Sanitation, Dr Jin Yinlong of China Centers for Disease Control, worked alongside the TWG WHS membership to obtain the data presented and discussed in this report.

Special mention should be made of the following national sector professionals for their important contribution to this work through the formulation of an analysis of the sanitation status in their respective countries. They are as follows: Brunei Darussalam: Abu Bakar bin Haji Awang Mohd Salleh; Abdullah Sani bin Aji; Abdul Mushawwir bin Abd Rahman; and, Young Chee Yeen; Cambodia: Chea Samnang; Mao Saray; and, Pen Saroeun; China: Jin Yinlong and Shunqing Xu; Indonesia: Sharad Adhikary; Handy Legowo; Abdul Mukti; Oswar Mungkasa; Zainal Nampira; M. Sholah Imari; and, Nugroho Tri Utomo; Japan: Hirokatsu Asakawa and Mari Asami; Lao PDR: Tayphasavanh Fengthong; Malaysia: Ir Zulkifli Tamby Chik; Izham Harith Ikhwan; Samah Che Lamin; Amad Mahmud Muslim; Sasitheran K. Nair; Dorai Narayana; Engku Azman Tuan Mat; Tauran Zaidi Ahmad Zaidi; and, Mohd Hanif Zailani; Mongolia: Altanzagas Badrakh; Ts. Badrakh; Tsetsegsaihan Batmunkh; I. Bolormaa; D. Myagmar; Oyunchimeg; Enkhstetseg Shinee; and, Tsedenbaljir; Republic of Korea: Chang¬gyun Jin; PanGyi Kim; and, Ji Hyun Lee; Singapore: Young Chee Yen; Philippines: Joselito Riego de Dios; Timor-Leste: Dinesh Bajracharya; Bishnu Prasad Pokhrel; Jesse Shapiro; and, Tomasia de Sousa; Viet Nam: Truong Dinh Bac and Tran Dac Phu.

Robert Bos and Khondkar Rifat Hossain of WHO Headquarters should be thanked for contributing the 2010 revised country sanitation coverage utilized in this report. Acknowledgement is also made of the support provided by Fiona Gore, also of WHO Headquarters, for providing the most recent WHO health statistics used in this document.

The suggestions on the draft document by Olivia Castillo, UNSGAB; Jan Willem Rosenboom and Richard Gross, of WSP/Cambodia; Shinee Enkhtsetseg of WHO/Mongolia; Tuan Nghia Ton of WHO/Viet Nam; Bonifacio Magtibay of WHO/Philippines; Lala Sihombing of Cambodia; and Zhenbo Yang of China, were greatly appreciated.

Special mention should be made of the overall support to this process by Terrence Thompson of WHO/WPRO.

Jose Hueb, WHO consultant, prepared the templates for country level data collection and drafted this report.

Alexander Pascual did the design and layout of the document. Raquel Amparo of WHO/WPRO provided effective administrative support to the development of this assessment.

The preparation of this report would not have been possible without the generous support of the United States Agency for International Development, which is gratefully acknowledged.

Photo credits: All images courtesy of WEDC. © Brian Skinner on page vi; © Rebecca Scott on pages x and 30; © Peter Harvey on page 4; © WEDC Photolibrary on pages 11, 21 and 37; © Darren Saywell (IWA) on pages 12, 42 and 50; © Brian Skinner on pages 13 and 28.

Preface

About 800 million people in East Asia still lack access today to improved sanitation facilities. This represents almost 40% of East Asia's population, which is devoid of this basic service and therefore affected repeatedly by crippling sanitation-related infirmities. This marginalized segment of the population, usually the poor living in rural areas and densely populated urban slums, is denied the fundamental human right of enjoying good health and fair opportunities for social and economic development.

Access to basic sanitation is being viewed increasingly as an essential human right and as a fundamental element of poverty alleviation, good health and economic growth. There is also a clear perception that investments to improve sanitation are urgently needed in East Asia if a sustained development process is to be attained in this Region, which comprises 16 countries of the South-East Asia and Eastern Asia regions.

The first East Asia Ministerial Conference on Sanitation and Hygiene (EASAN 2007) was held in Beppu City, Japan, from 30 November to 1 December 2007. The major outcome of this event was the Beppu Declaration, adopted by consensus by the heads of delegations of 13 countries.

The conference recognized that sustainable access to sanitation, in combination with practising hygienic behaviour, is fundamental to the achievement of many other Millennium Development Goals (MDG) to which the participating governments have committed. It was acknowledged that access to basic sanitation and safe water supply and good hygienic behaviour are necessary for the health and well-being of the population and are fundamental in order for people to live in dignity and safety.

The conference also recognized that the governments of East Asian countries approved the Charter of the Regional Forum on Environment and Health in August 2007 in Bangkok, Thailand, and the work plans of six regional thematic working groups, including the one on water supply, hygiene and sanitation, and that this is bound to a vision of universal sanitation and good hygiene in the Region.

Despite major efforts and impressive achievements, the sanitation challenge in the Region remains daunting: if the coverage trend of the past 18 years continues to 2015, the MDG sanitation target of 74% will be missed by six percentage points. Projections indicate that by 2015, one-third of the population still will not be served. And even if the MDG sanitation target is achieved, about 600 million people in this Region will witness the arrival of 2015 without access to improved sanitation.

The second East Asia Ministerial Conference on Sanitation and Hygiene (EASAN2) heralds a significant opportunity to improve international mechanisms to advance the sanitation and hygiene agenda in the Region. With the participation at EASAN2 of the Thematic Working Group on Water, Hygiene and Sanitation (TWG WHS), it will be possible to discuss mechanisms to streamline strategic approaches and action for sanitation development in the Region.

EASAN 2007 identified the constraints for sanitation and hygiene improvement, established a firm commitment to remove such barriers and set the tone for regional and national action. It is expected that the second conference in Manila in January 2010 will reach far beyond what already has been achieved. There is a need to streamline international action, make it a dynamic mechanism to support individual Member States in formulating their sanitation agenda and convert regional findings and recommendations into effective planning, programming and financing of the sanitation sector in each developing East Asian country.

Executive summary

> "Lack of sanitation breeds the so-called diseases of filth. These are diseases caused by the faecal contamination of food, water, or soil, or spread by flies that feed on filth. In the absence of sanitation, huge numbers of people are, in effect, being sickened by ingestion of infected excrement. This is intolerable amidst the collective wealth of the 21st century". Margaret Chan, WHO Director General, World Water Day, 2008.

The main objective of this document is to provide an overview of the status of sanitation in East Asia to support decisions and recommendations in light of the collective governments' commitments expressed in the Beppu Declaration on 1 December 2007. The countries included in this analysis are those in the East Asia Region.

Three information sources were used to prepare this document: information from a template completed by most East Asian countries; data on access to sanitation services from the new revision of coverage statistics from WHO and UNICEF Joint Monitoring Programme for Water Supply and Sanitation (JMP); and literature by different authors describing sanitation concepts and experiences at country level.

According to country statistics provided by the JMP database updated in 2010, the proportion of people served with some type of improved sanitation in East Asia rose from 48% in 1990 to 62% in 2008. This means that despite a total population growth of 20% over the same period, the proportion of people in the Region served with sanitation increased 14 percentage points. Despite this major effort, about two of every five people in East Asia are still without access to improved sanitation.

Almost 500 million additional people in East Asia received access to an improved sanitation facility between 1990 and 2008. Despite this major improvement, almost 300 million people still need to share an improved type of sanitation facility with other households, whereas nearly 400 million use precarious unimproved facilities and over 100 million simply defecate in the open. The rural population without access to sanitation services in East Asia is almost half a billion people, which is over 60% more than the 300 million urban dwellers unserved.

The Region is not on track to achieve the MDG sanitation target. It will fall short by 6% of the MDG sanitation regional target of 74% by 2015. It is likely that even if the target is achieved, there will remain major challenges to synchronize people's needs with environmental and health requirements.

Not surprisingly, diarrhoeal diseases are a major killer in this Region. They are largely preventable by good sanitation and hygiene and a sufficient and safe water supply. Improved sanitation alone reduces diarrhoea death rates by a third (UNICEF, WHO, 2009). In East Asia, there are 450 million cases of diarrhoea every year and the number of deaths reaches nearly 150 000 a year (WHO, 2008a). Estimates suggest that the overall incidence of diarrhoeal diseases has remained relatively stable over the past two decades whereas the death rate has decreased consistently. This indicates that while case management approaches and practises improve over time, the preventive aspects (good sanitation, hygiene, safe drinking-water, food safety) are not progressing as effectively.

Despite the rather negative analysis, there has been remarkable progress in sanitation in East Asia since the 1990 baseline year. Increasing coverage by 14 percentage points in 18 years during a period of huge population growth proves that much greater progress can be achieved should East Asian countries be more committed to improving sanitation in the Region.

One of the major drawbacks in the Region is a lack of good information about sanitation and water systems that could provide sound analyses for national policy-making, planning and programming. Generally, the national information systems, where they exist, are not well integrated into national planning.

As for hygiene, most countries perceive the effectiveness of their hygiene education programmes as normal within a scale that ranges from excellent to very poor. All countries reported the existence of a national strategy or plan to promote sanitation but half of them indicated that this is not being implemented fully. Most of the countries reported that hygiene behaviour is not included effectively in the primary or secondary school curricula. The primary recommendation is the need to create awareness among policy-makers about the importance of hygiene promotion and formulation and putting into effect a national plan in this regard.

A major finding of this survey is that information about financial investments, past and future, either does not exist or is unavailable. Given the absence of country-level information about finance, policy-making and strategic planning will continue to be conducted based either on inaccurate assumptions or on international estimates of expenditures.

While sanitation coverage statistics suggest a dire situation, several countries reported important sanitation interventions that might help improve things in the near future. Typical examples are the Community-Based Total Sanitation in Indonesia (CBTS), the National Programme for Sanitation Facilities in Mongolia, the National Sanitation Roadmap in the Philippines and the National Target Programme for Rural Water Supply and Sanitation in Viet Nam. China is implementing its National Urban Hygiene and Sanitation "Eleventh Five-Year Plan", which is its national plan for hygiene and sanitation.

There is emerging awareness in the Region that a shift in sanitation financing is required from financing "subsidies and grants for sanitation facilities" to the poor to funding "sanitation promotion and leveraging resources". Most countries reported well-structured initiatives to generate sanitation demand through social marketing using different methodologies. Community-led sanitation programmes appear to have attracted the attention of decision-makers in several countries, where this approach is under way experimentally or has been put into effect completely.

Most countries consider that the participation of women, children and poor families and the public and private sectors in planning and implementing sanitation programmes is insufficient. Just one country – the Lao People's Democratic Republic – responded that it was sufficient.

Very few respondents to the TWG WHS template reported effective action to stimulate local governments to play a more active role in sanitation improvement. This is consistent with the view that most countries consider that both local governments and local private sectors have sanitation staffs that are largely untrained and unprepared to deal with this important issue. But most countries reported effective action at national levels to bridge such a gap.

Country responses to the TWG WHS templates indicate that the information available on the status of sanitation in public primary or secondary schools is remarkably weak. There is usually no monitoring system in place to measure the availability and quality of sanitation services in these facilities. The few lower income countries reporting about this indicated a relatively low level of hygienic sanitation facilities functioning in primary or secondary schools, which ranges from 12% in Viet Nam to 78% in Cambodia. With regard to health care establishments, this number ranges from 30% in Mongolia to 80% in China.

Responsibilities for sanitation, especially rural sanitation, are not clearly defined in most East Asian countries and are somehow an afterthought in different national or local agencies. Responsibilities for sanitation and communication and coordination mechanisms among agencies appear to be blurred in most countries and in some cases simply do not exist. A crucial recommendation is the urgent need to establish a clear national institutional framework for sanitation, including the definition of roles and responsibilities of different national and subnational stakeholders.

When asked about constraints to sanitation improvement, respondents indicated that the primary issues include a lack of coordination mechanisms to synchronize rural sanitation action, poor operation and maintenance, lack of community awareness about hygiene and sanitation, insufficient financial resources for construction and operation of sanitation facilities and the lack of priority given to sanitation in national development plans.

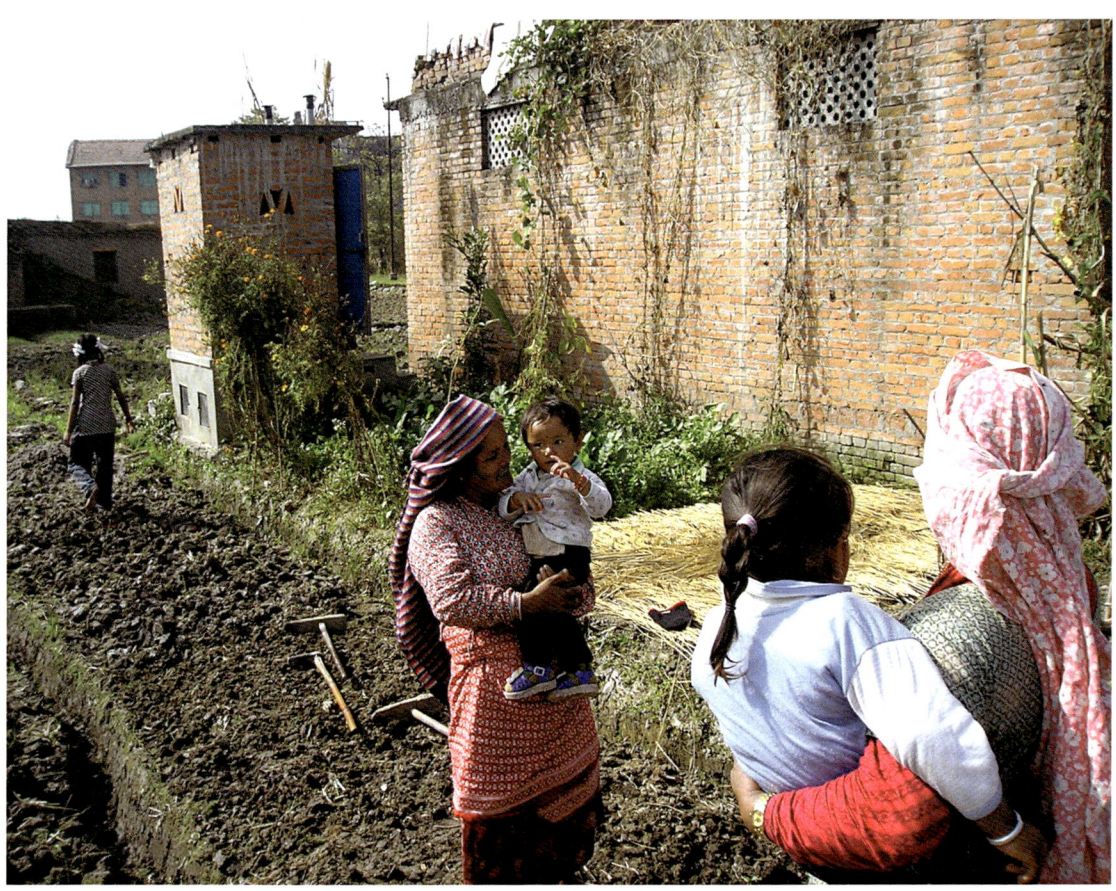

How to solve the sanitation problem? Respondents to the TWG WHS template provided a wealth of recommendations about policies and strategies, institutional and legal issues, financing, monitoring and evaluation and capacity-building. The common denominator of these recommendations is the need to organize effectively the institutional frameworks at the national level and establish sound financial mechanisms that would allow effective planning, programming, implementation and monitoring of action to improve sanitation.

If the trend continues towards coverage projections showing that the MDG sanitation target will be missed by 6 percentage points by 2015, then achieving universal coverage appears to be out of reach in East Asia. If the trends are to be maintained, universal coverage will not be achieved in rural areas before another 40 years and in urban areas it only will be achieved 90 years from now. Urgent action is needed to reverse this trend, as proposed by the East Asian countries themselves throughout this document.

When asked what could be done to enhance the cooperation and exchange of information among East Asian countries, respondents indicated they would like to see greater involvement of the Region in global exchanges on sanitation, more frequent meetings of East Asian countries for increased exchange of information, regionally organized training workshops, more effective exchange of information, networking and joint regional project preparation and implementation. Achieving this will require that EASAN moves from a mere biennial regional forum to an instrument that will convert these national desires into action. This document provides different scenarios to stimulate discussion about strengthening and making operational the EASAN Platform, including the formation of a steering committee and a secretariat responsible for putting into effect action agreed upon at EASAN forums.

Introduction

Three major information sources were used to prepare this document. The first came from a template containing questions addressing the commitments expressed in the Beppu Declaration (Annex I), which was sent to the 14 East Asian nations represented at the TWG WHS. The responses to these questions, provided by 13 countries (Brunei Darussalam, Cambodia, China, Indonesia, Japan, the Lao People's Democratic Republic, Malaysia, Mongolia, the Philippines, the Republic of Korea, Singapore, Timor-Leste and Viet Nam) formed a wealth of information used for the sanitation sector analysis contained in this report. It is important to highlight that the accuracy of the information in this report is directly linked to the quality of information provided by the responders to the templates at country level.

A second source of information refers basically to data about access to sanitation services from the WHO and UNICEF JMP statistical update referred to 2008. Most of the analyses about access to sanitation services were based on JMP statistics rather than on those reported by the TWG WHS membership. The reason was that the latter information does not allow comparison among countries because the definition of adequate sanitation varies from country to country and does not allow the analysis of coverage trends.

The third source is literature on sanitation by different authors that describes concepts and experiences at country level.

The whole East Asia Region was considered in this analysis: Brunei Darussalam, The Democratic People's Republic of Korea, Cambodia, China, Indonesia, Japan, The Lao People's Democratic Republic, Malaysia, Mongolia, Myanmar, The Philippines, The Republic of Korea, Singapore, Thailand, Timor-Leste, Viet Nam.

By no means is this document intended to replace more comprehensive national sanitation, hygiene and water sector assessments being undertaken globally or in different countries of this Region.

An immense desire and outstanding efforts to advance the sanitation agenda in East Asia are described throughout this report. Despite such efforts and the extraordinary economic growth in the Region, about one-third of the population still lacks access to improved sanitation. Inadequate sanitation and poor hygiene are major causes of disease and deprivation, perpetuate the circle of poverty and exacerbate the gap between the wealthy and the poor.

A major achievement of EASAN conferences is to provide a platform to discuss options for accelerated national action on sanitation, taking into account gloomy sanitation trends, the dire status of the sector and how to streamline different initiatives in the Region that deal with this fundamental subject.

Background

This decade witnessed initiatives worldwide to emphasize the importance of sanitation to health and economic growth and to elicit firm commitments for better sanitation at the highest possible political levels in both poor and emerging nations as well as in more advanced countries. The visible portion of these efforts was a series of ministerial conferences to address this issue. Country-level action continues to unfold less visibly but conspicuously impacts the sector locally as we approach 2015, the critical date for the achievement of the MDG sanitation target.

The World Summit on Sustainable Development (WSSD), held in Johannesburg, South Africa, from 26 August to 4 September 2002, marked a major cornerstone in international sanitation improvement. It was decided that sanitation should be included as part of the MDGs formulated in 2000 at the Millennium Summit. Another major achievement, in recognition of the growing importance of sanitation and hygiene on the international agenda, was the declaration by the United Nations General Assembly of 2008 as the International Year of Sanitation.

Important regional initiatives during this decade, specifically on sanitation, include: the African Conference on Sanitation (AfricaSan), Johannesburg, South Africa, in 2002; AfricaSan+5, in Durban, South Africa, in 2008; the South Asian Conference on Sanitation (SACOSAN), in Dhaka, Bangladesh, in October 2003; SACOSAN II, in Islamabad, Pakistan, in September 2006; SACOSAN III in New Delhi, India, in October 2008; the First Latin American Conference on Sanitation (LatinoSan) in Cali, Colombia, in November 2007; and the First East Asia Ministerial Conference on Sanitation and Hygiene (EASAN), in Beppu City, Japan, in November 2007.

A crucial resolution of EASAN was the creation of a regional platform for cooperation in sanitation and hygiene, which included an East Asia Ministerial Conference on Sanitation and Hygiene to be held in the Region, provisionally biennially, building preferably on existing forums and facilitating cooperation among East Asian countries and between this Region and other regions of the world (WHO, WSP, UNICEF, 2008).

Another significant milestone in Asia in 2007 was the First Ministerial Regional Forum on Environment and Health in Southeast and Eastern Asian countries held in Bangkok, Thailand, in August of that year. The general objective of this Regional initiative is to deal effectively with environmental health problems within and among countries by increasing the capacity of Southeast and East Asian countries to deal with environmental health management (WHO, UNEP, 2007). The regional forum decided to establish a TWG WHS along with another five thematic working groups covering different environmental health issues. Knowledge management, technical support, coordination and advocacy and resource mobilization are among the top priorities of this group.

Objectives of this document

- To provide an overview of the status of sanitation in East Asia to support decisions and recommendations at EASAN2 held in Manila, Philippines, from 27 to 29 January 2010;
- To take stock of major initiatives addressing sanitation in the Region and reflect on ways to streamline international efforts;
- To assess the formulation of sanitation action in East Asian countries in light of the collective governments' commitments as expressed in the Beppu Declaration on 1 December 2007; and
- To provide the basis for discussion and intensive advocacy work at all levels to accelerate investment in the improvement of sanitation and hygiene in East Asia.

Target audience

This report provides relevant information on sanitation and hygiene addressing most of the East Asian countries to support decisions relating to investment, planning, management and quality of service in the sector, primarily to be used as a source of information for EASAN2. It is also prepared for those who want information about where the sanitation sector stands in the Region and how it is changing over time. These include national government policy- and decision-makers, planners and consultants, bilateral and multilateral agency staff, researchers and overall sector professionals throughout the Region.

Demography and health

Population

The population of East Asia experienced intensive urbanization and a steady reduction in rural population during the period 1990-2008. Although the population of the Region is still predominantly rural, such a status will be reversed by 2015 (Figure 1). The total population of the Region accounts for over 30% of the world population.

FIGURE 1   Urban and rural population of East Asia, 1990, 2008 and 2015 (projected)

As an average, every single day, East Asia sees the emergence of 62 thousand new urban citizens. This means that just keeping up with the current level of sanitation services, basic urban infrastructure needs to be provided daily to a new population equivalent to that of a sizeable town.

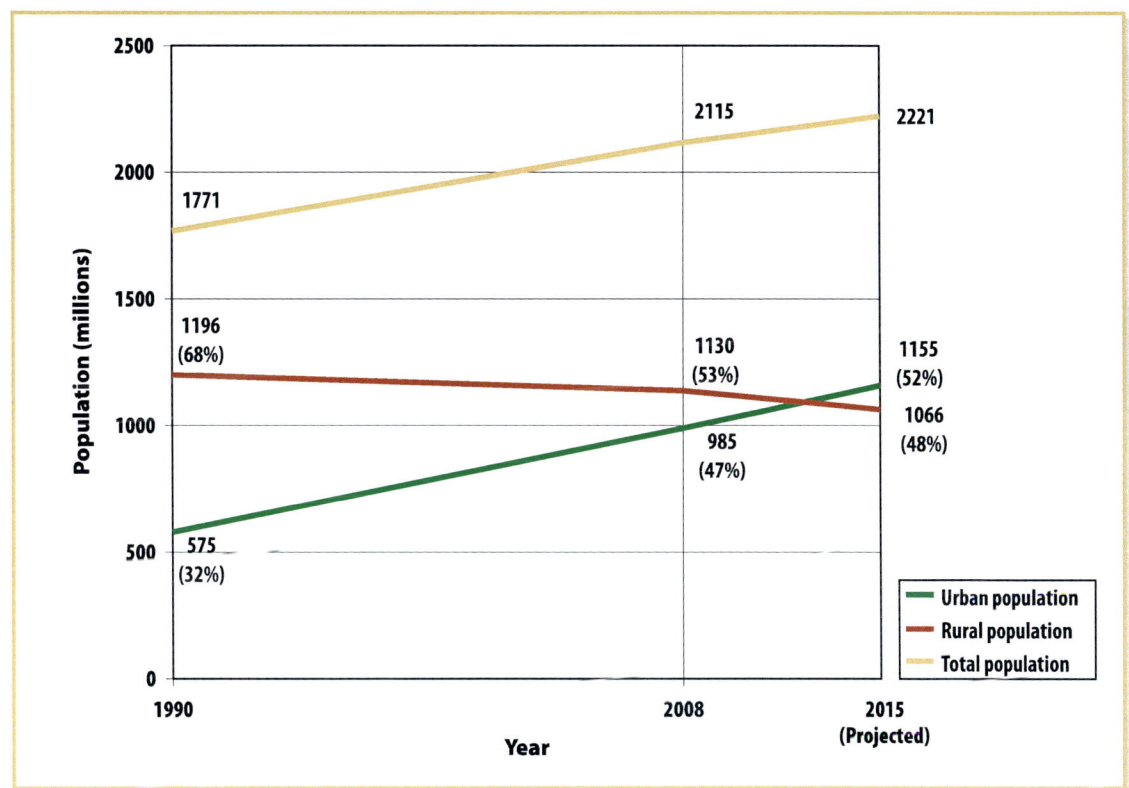

Source: Country population from UNPD (2009)

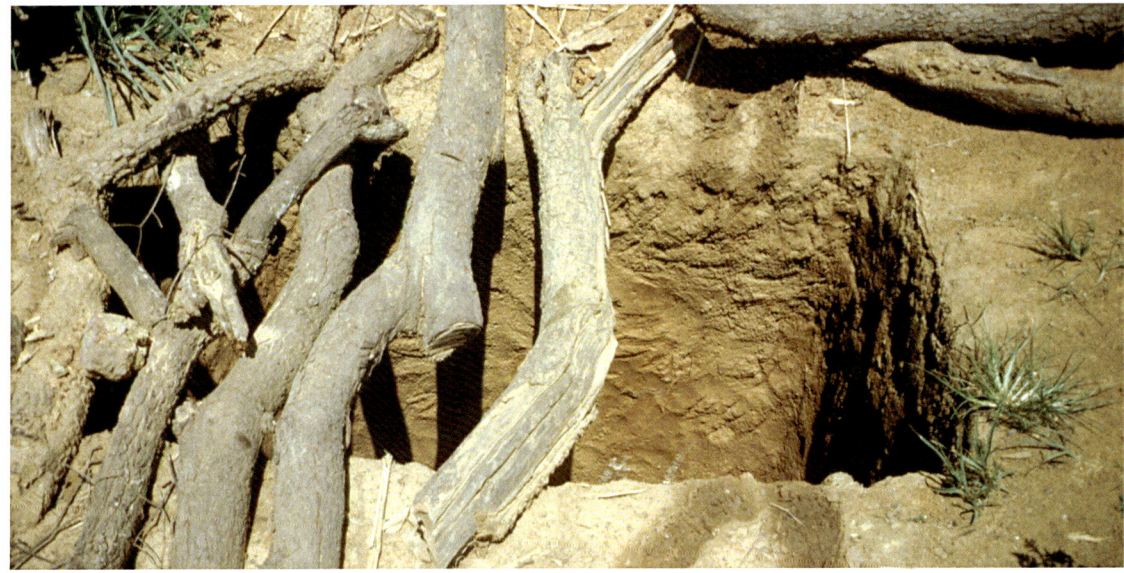

Health

Infectious and parasitic diseases remain the major killers of children in developing countries (WHO, 2003). Although notable success has been achieved in certain areas, diarrhoeal diseases still represent the second biggest cause of child deaths in most East Asian countries (Figure 2).

Mortality of children under 5 years old is closely related to access to basic sanitation and safe drinking-water, as demonstrated in numerous

FIGURE 2 Distribution of causes of death among children under 5 years old in East Asian countries

Diarrhoeal diseases are the second biggest cause of mortality among children under 5 years old in over 60% of the countries in East Asia.

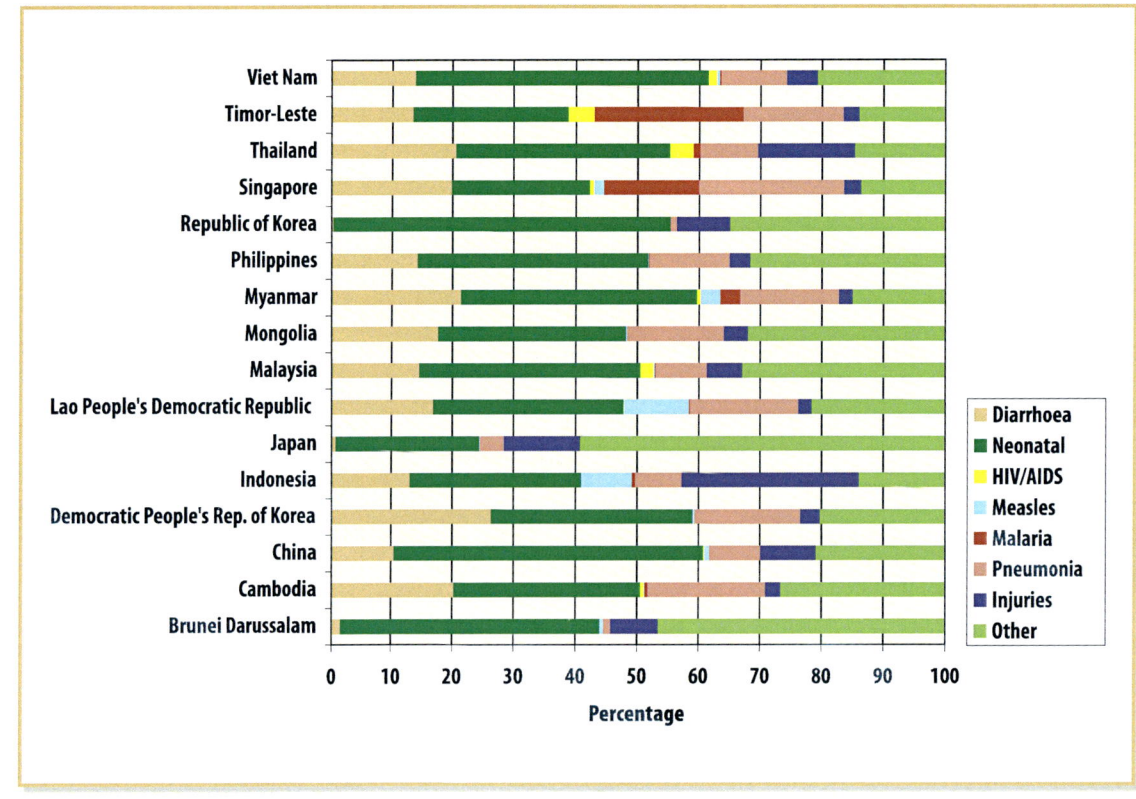

Source: Country statistics from WHO (2009)

research projects worldwide. Remarkable progress has been made during the period 1990-2007 in East Asian countries in reducing under-five mortality, with over one-third of the countries reducing their under-five mortality rate to less than a half of the values of 1990 (Figure 3). Improved sanitation services, better hygiene behaviour and access to safe drinking-water, especially by mothers, are crucial in reducing child mortality and extending the life expectancy of children.

Diarrhoeal diseases often are described as water-related but more accurately should be known as excreta-related since the pathogens derive from faecal matter. This may enter the mouth via contaminated drinking-water but can equally come from dirty hands, unwashed raw food, utensils or smears on clothes (UN-Water, 2008).

While there are numerous diarrhoea-causing organisms, the majority of cases in virtually all settings are caused by the following organisms: viruses (rotavirus); bacteria (enterotoxigenic *Escherichia coli*, *Shigella*, *Campylobacter jeuni*, *Vibrio cholerae*, Salmonella (non-typhoid), Enteropathogenic *Escherichia coli*); protozoa (Cryptosporidium) (WHO, 1999).

FIGURE 3 Under-five mortality rate per 1000 live births in East Asian countries, 1990 and 2007

Although progress has been made in East Asian countries in reducing under-five mortality between 1990 and 2007, there are still huge disparities between countries presenting the highest and the lowest mortality rates.

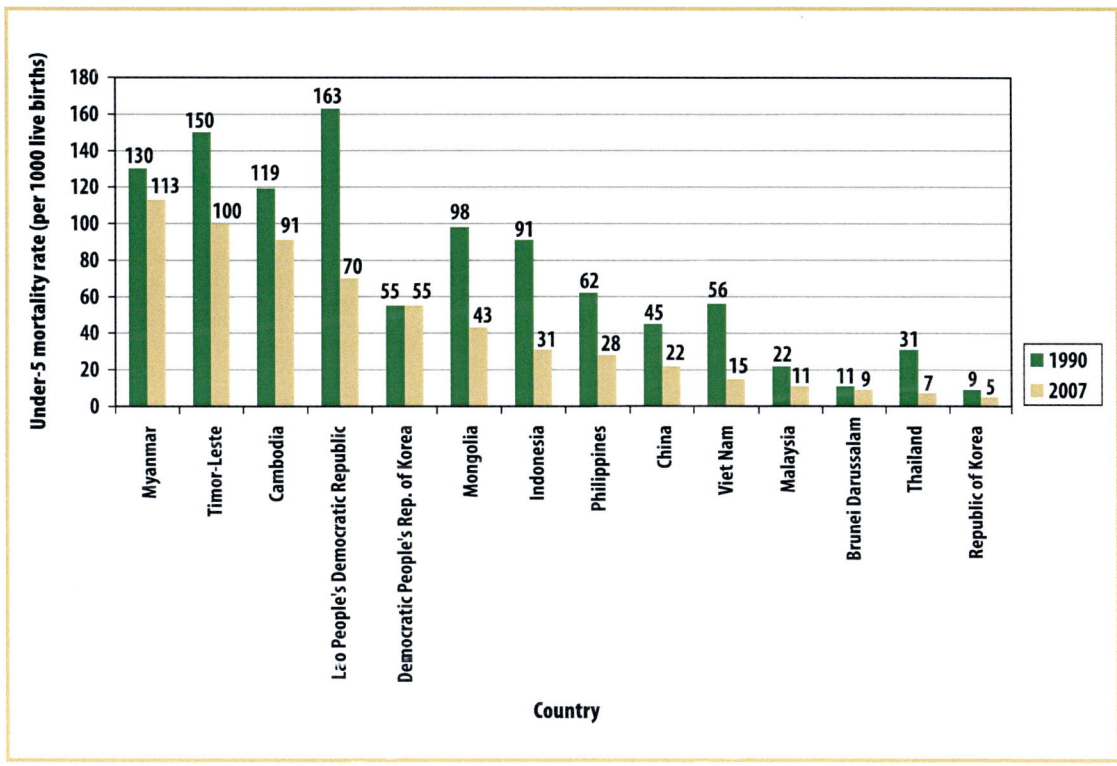

Source: Country statistics from WHO (2009)

Figure 4 indicates the pathways of contamination of humans through "waves" of contamination. From the primary sources of contamination (human and animal excreta, animal products), the contamination cascades through different routes to humans, who contract different types of sanitation-related diseases, including cholera and other epidemic diarrhoeal diseases. For each of these routes there is a need to create barriers

diarrhoea every year and the number of deaths due to diarrhoeal diseases reaches nearly 150 000 a year (WHO, 2008a) (Figures 5 and 6). Fully 88% of cases of diarrhoeal diseases worldwide are attributable to inadequate sanitation, unsafe water and poor hygiene (Prüss-Üstün A et al., 2008). Improved sanitation reduces diarrhoea death rates by a third (UNICEF, WHO, 2009). Estimates suggest that the overall incidence

FIGURE 4 "Waves" of human contamination from human excreta, animal excreta and animal products

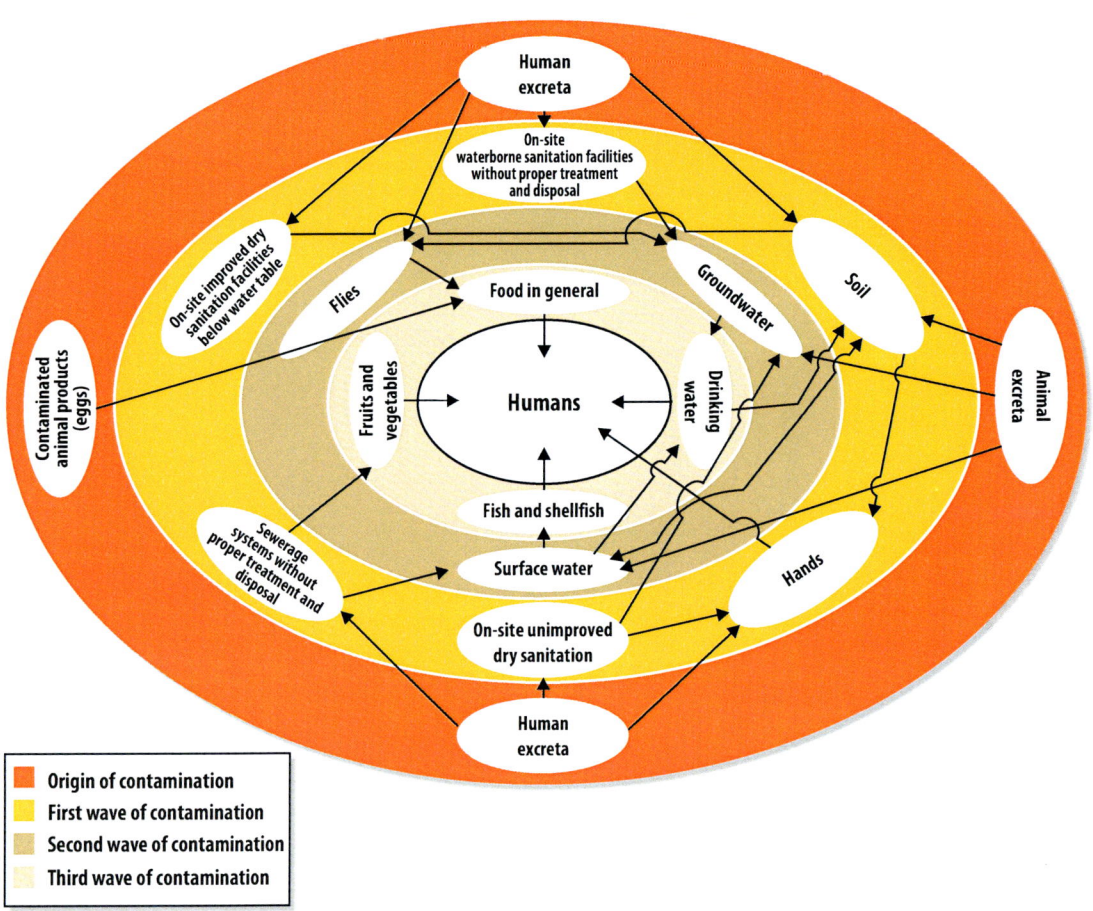

Source: Adapted from WHO/Western Pacific Regional Office (2008), Prüss-Üstün A et al. (2008) and Wagner KG, Lanoix JN (1958).

to prevent contamination from reaching the next level. The use of good hygienic sanitation facilities and hand washing are the most crucial contamination barriers.

At the same time that diarrhoeal diseases are a major killer, they also largely are preventable. In East Asia, there are 450 million cases of

of diarrhoeal diseases has remained relatively stable over the past two decades whereas the death rate has decreased consistently. This is an indication that while case management approaches and practises are improving over time, the preventive aspects (good sanitation, hygiene, drinking-water, food safety) are not progressing as effectively.

FIGURE 5   Annual incidence rates of diarrhoeal diseases per 1000 population in the East Asian countries, 2004

Nearly half of the countries in East Asia have an annual incidence rate of diarrhoeal diseases above 400 cases per 1 000 population.

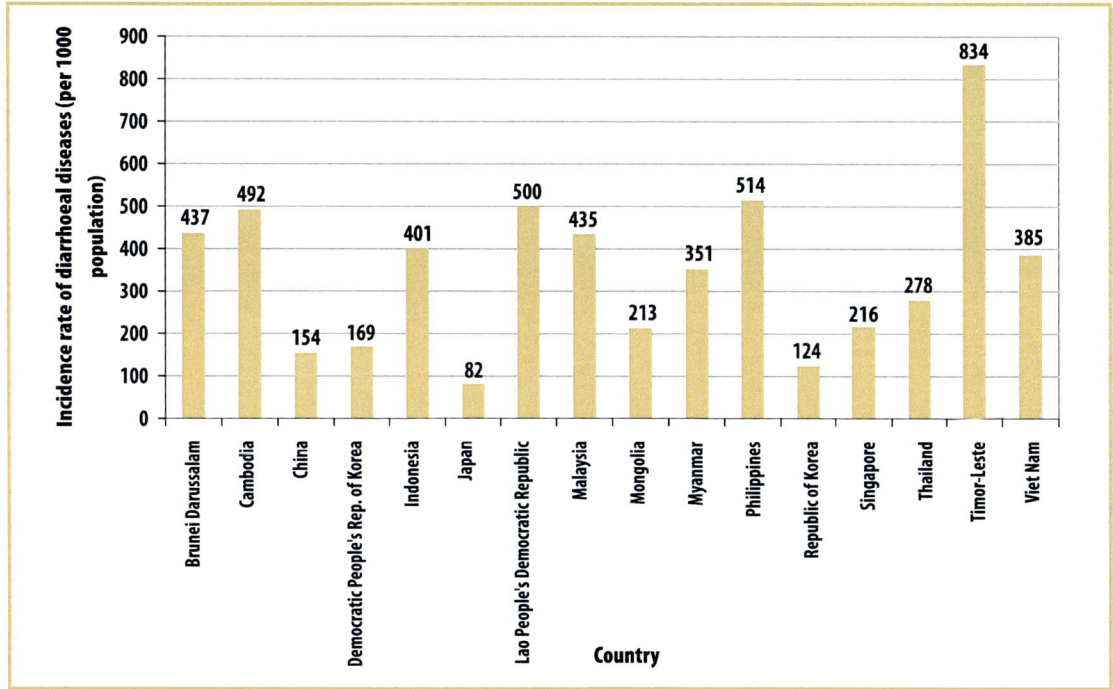

Source: Country statistics from WHO (2008)

FIGURE 6   Deaths due to diarrhoeal diseases per 100 000 population in the East Asian countries in 2004

Six countries managed to keep the death rate due to diarrhoeal diseases below five per 100 000 people. Two countries have rates of about 40 deaths per 100 000.

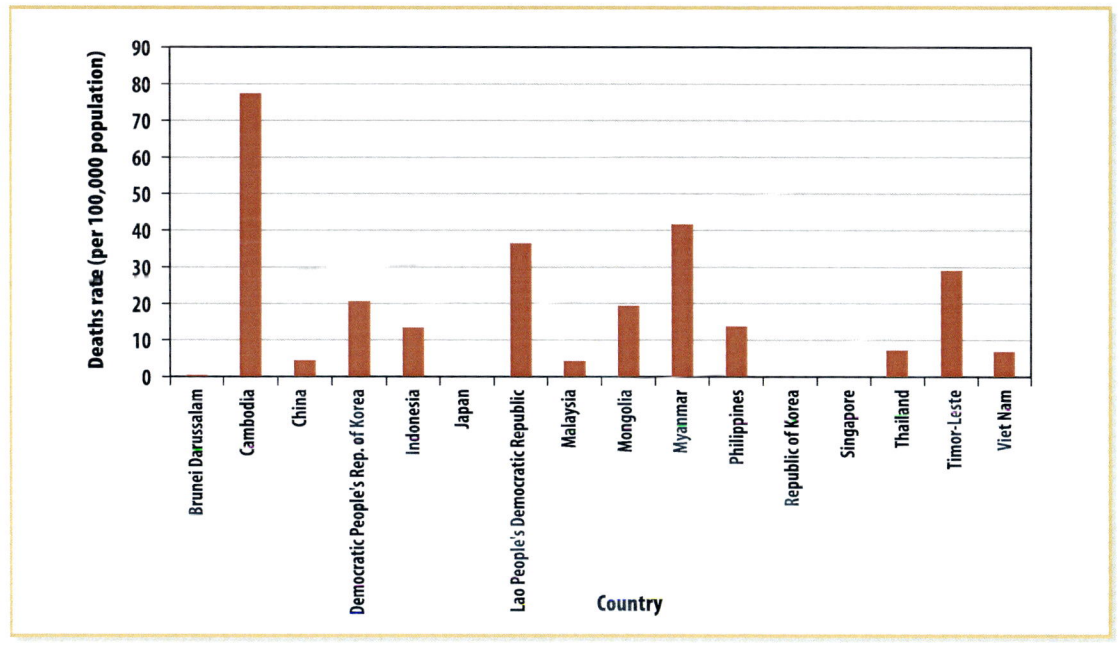

Source: Country statistics from WHO (2008)

TABLE 1 Groups of sanitation categories

Groups of sanitation categories according to the JMP	Categories of services	Grouping according to the MDG definition of improved sanitation
Improved sanitation facilities*	Flush or pour-flush to: • piped sewer system • septic tank • pit latrine Ventilated improved pit latrine (VIP) Pit latrine with slab Composting toilet	Improved
Sharing improved sanitation facilities	Same as above but shared by one or more households.	
Unimproved sanitation facilities (other unimproved)	Flush or pour-flush to elsewhere** Pit latrine without slab or open pit Bucket latrine Hanging toilet or hanging latrine No facilities or bush or field (open defecation)	Unimproved
Open defecation	Absence of sanitation facilities.	

* Only facilities that are not shared or public are considered improved.
** Excreta are flushed to the street, yard or plot, open sewer, a ditch and a drainage way.
Source: Based on WHO, UNICEF (2008)

Status of sanitation

Definition of sanitation

There is widespread agreement internationally on the definition of sanitation by the United Nations Millennium Project Task Force on Water and Sanitation (2005): basic sanitation is the lowest-cost option for securing sustainable access to safe, hygienic and convenient facilities and services for excreta and sullage disposal that provides privacy and dignity while ensuring a clean and healthful living environment both at home and in the neighbourhood of users. Although this is conceptually sound, it is not feasible to monitor access to sanitation services based on such a definition because most of the elements within this formulation are not included in existing household surveys.

For this reason, the JMP uses a proxy to basic sanitation. The assumption is that the types of sanitation facilities categorized as "improved" are more likely to fulfil the requirements of a "basic" sanitation facility than the "unimproved" ones (Table 2).

The JMP is the United Nations mechanism tasked with monitoring progress towards the MDG drinking-water and sanitation target. In fulfilling this mandate, the JMP publishes updated estimates every two years on the various types of drinking water sources and sanitation facilities being used worldwide (WHO, UNICEF, 2008) (Box 1).

Indicator definitions and population estimates used by the JMP may differ from those used by national governments. This is illustrated in subsequent sections of this report.

For each report published by the JMP, the country, regional and global estimates on access to water supply and sanitation facilities are revised. Such changes may include the recalculation of 1990 baseline coverage statistics. For this reason, the data published in successive JMP reports are not comparable (WHO, UNICEF, 2008). However, an outstanding feature of the JMP's statistics is that values concerning the same indicators can be compared among countries because they are

BOX 1 WHO and UNICEF Joint Monitoring Programme for Water Supply and Sanitation (JMP)

The statistics used to monitor progress on the use of improved sanitation and dinking-water in each country and globally are produced by the JMP. This is the official mechanism adopted by the United Nations Secretary General and the entire United Nations System to report on progress in the provision of improved sanitation and drinking-water services to the world population.

Since 2000, the JMP's coverage statistics are based on household surveys including: USAID-supported Demographic and Health Surveys (DHS); UNICEF-supported Multiple Indicator Cluster Surveys (MICS); national census reports; WHO-supported World Health Surveys; and other reliable national surveys that allow data to be compared. Household survey information give a much clearer comparison between countries, as they record the percentage of people using well defined improved facilities, as determined by face-to-face interviews.

Prior to the adoption of household surveys in 2000 as the basis for coverage reporting, coverage data were provided by the water utilities and ministries in charge of drinking-water and sanitation services. National definitions of "safe water" and "basic sanitation" differ widely from region to region and country to country, which makes it impossible to compare or aggregate official national coverage information into regional or global analyses.

The JMP's website (www.wssinfo.org) has an updated database of coverage statistics for most countries. The data are analysed biennially and presented in a global report.

Source: WHO, UNICEF (2005)

based on the same definition and referred to the same year.

Access to sanitation facilities

According to country statistics provided by the JMP database updated in 2010, the proportion of people served with some type of improved sanitation in East Asia rose from 48% in 1990 to 62% in 2008 (Figure 7). Despite the total population growth of 20% over the last 18 years, the proportion of people served with sanitation in the Region experienced an increase of coverage of 14 percentage points during the same period. Despite this major effort, about two of every five people in East Asia still do not have any type of improved sanitation facility.

Although there has been a small reduction in the proportion of people practising open defecation, it is still practised by over 130 million people throughout the countries of the Region.

FIGURE 7   Proportion of the East Asia population using an improved, shared or other unimproved sanitation facility or practising open defecation, 1990, 2008

Despite a major effort to increase sanitation coverage over the last 18 years, about two of every five people in East Asia still are not served with a private improved sanitation facility.

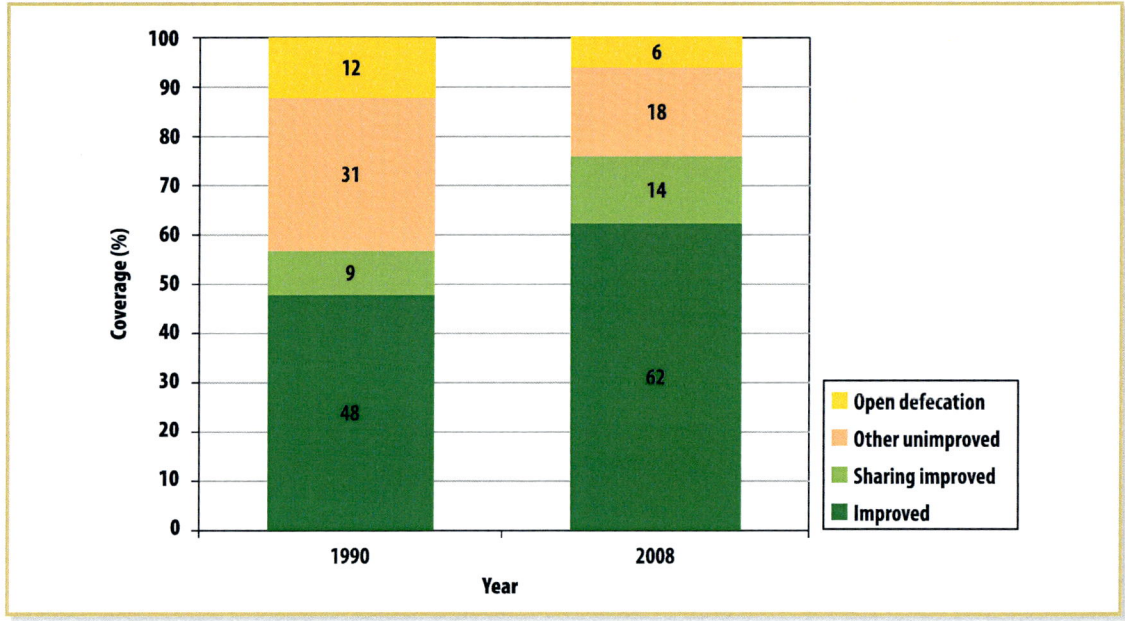

Source: Compiled from country coverage data from WHO and UNICEF JMP database.

Only half of the countries in East Asia have access to improved sanitation exceeding 60%. For the remaining seven countries, the coverage reaches values as low as 29% (Cambodia) and about 50% (Indonesia, the Lao People's Democratic Republic, Mongolia and Timor-Leste) (Figure 8).

FIGURE 8   Proportion of the population in East Asian countries using an improved, shared or other unimproved sanitation facility or practising open defecation, 2008

The Region presents a considerable disparity in access to improved sanitation, ranging from less than 30% (Cambodia) to universal coverage (Singapore, Republic of Korea and Japan). Open defecation is still widely practised in most countries.

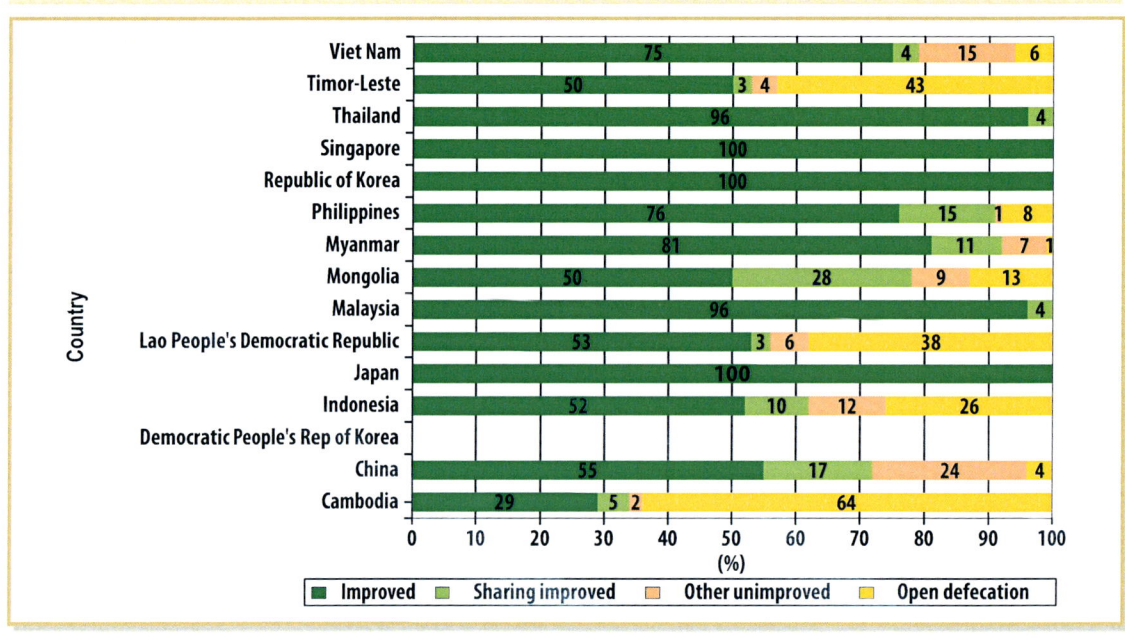

Source: Compiled from country coverage data from WHO and UNICEF JMP database

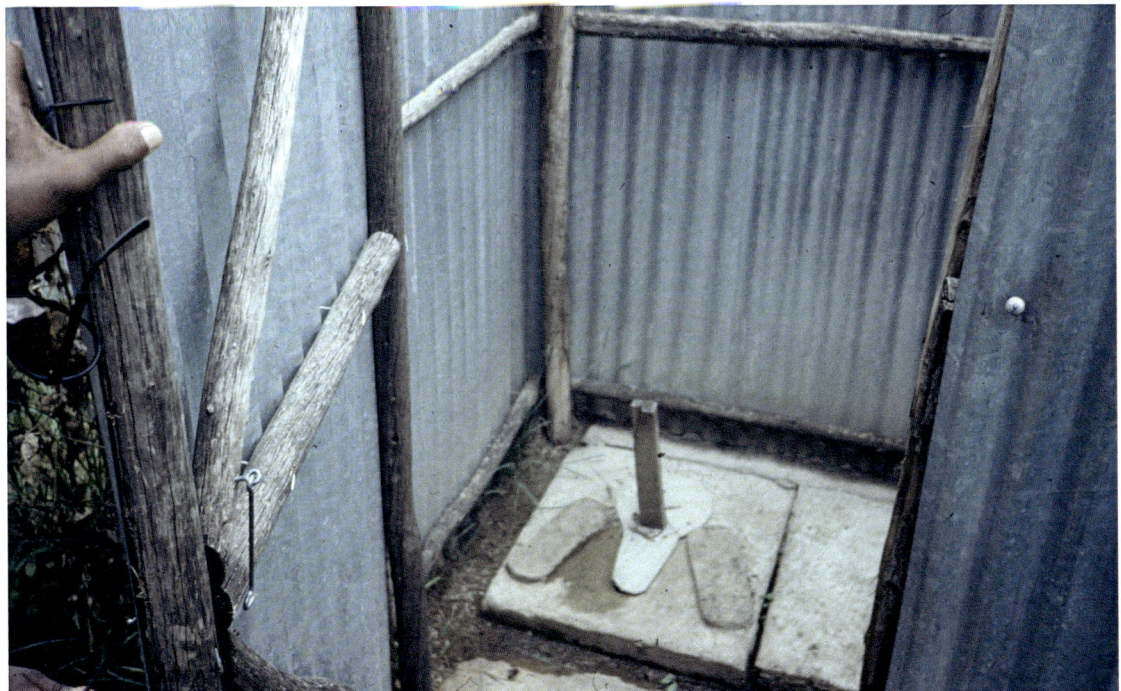

Almost 500 million additional people in East Asia received access to an improved sanitation facility between 1990 and 2008. Despite this major improvement, almost 300 million people still need to share an improved type of sanitation facility with other households. Nearly 400 million use precarious unimproved facilities and more than 130 million defecate in the open (Figure 9).

FIGURE 9 Population in East Asia using an improved, shared or other unimproved sanitation facility or practising open defecation, 1990, 2008

Between 1990 and 2008, more than 70 000 new people a day in East Asia received access to an improved sanitation facility, a remarkable achievement. However, the number of those not served is still exceedingly high, amounting to 800 million in 2008.

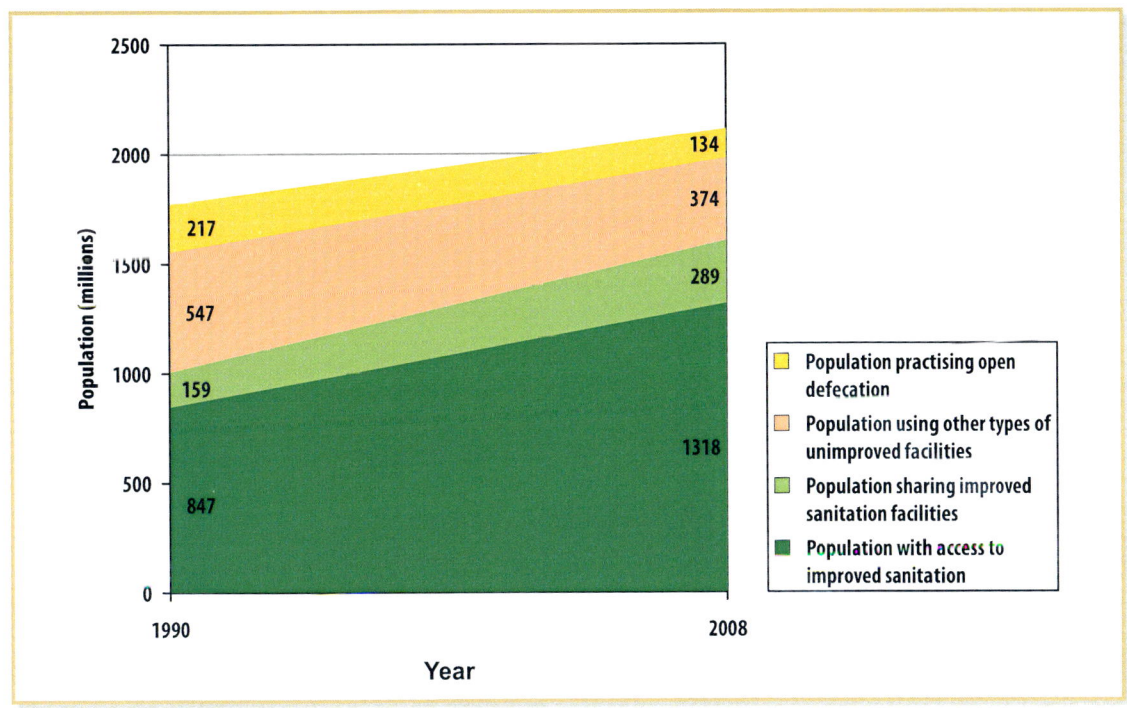

Source: Compiled from country coverage data from WHO and UNICEF JMP database

FIGURE 10 Urban and rural proportions of people with access to improved sanitation in East Asian countries, 2008

The countries in the Region that have lowest overall improved sanitation coverage are the same displaying a huge urban/rural coverage disparity (Cambodia, Indonesia, the Lao People's Democratic Republic, Mongolia, Timor-Leste and Viet Nam).

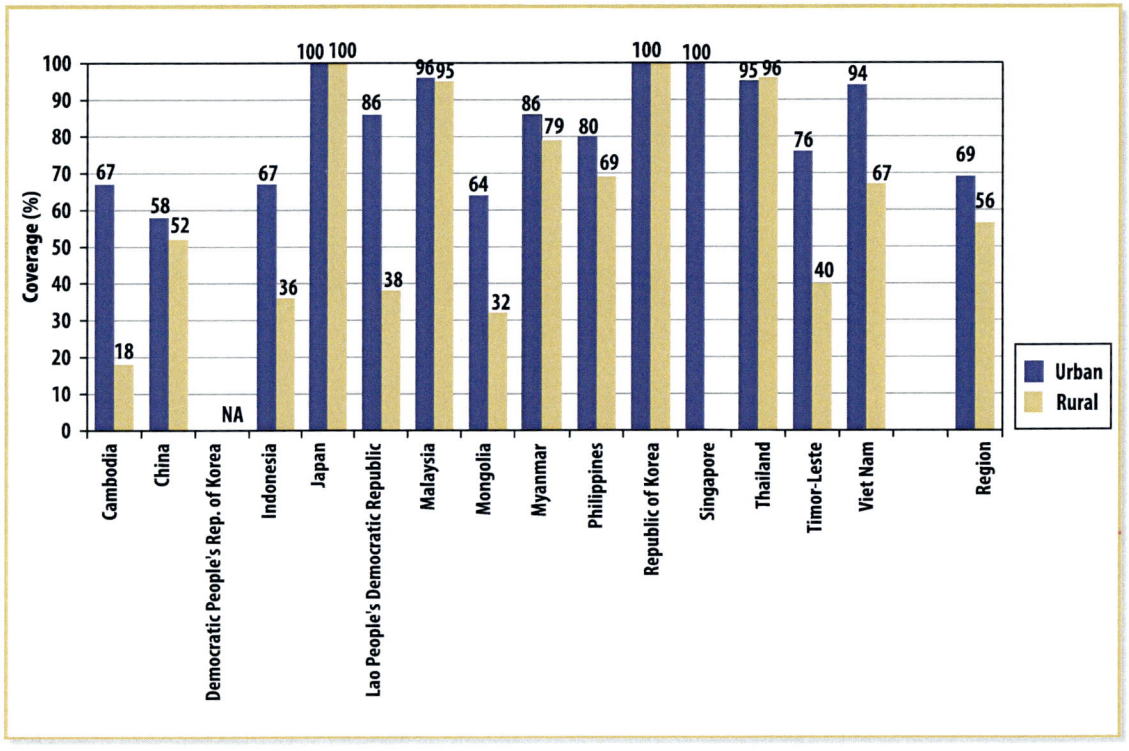

Source: Compiled from country coverage data from WHO and UNICEF JMP database

Trends in urban and rural coverage

Three countries of the Region (Cambodia, the Lao People's Democratic Republic and Mongolia) have doubled the improved sanitation coverage in urban areas than they do in rural areas (Figure 10). In addition to the high disparity in access to improved sanitation services between urban and rural areas, especially in countries of low total coverage, urban sanitation services are normally of a higher standard. While flushing toilets predominate in urban areas, most people in rural areas use outside dry sanitation facilities.

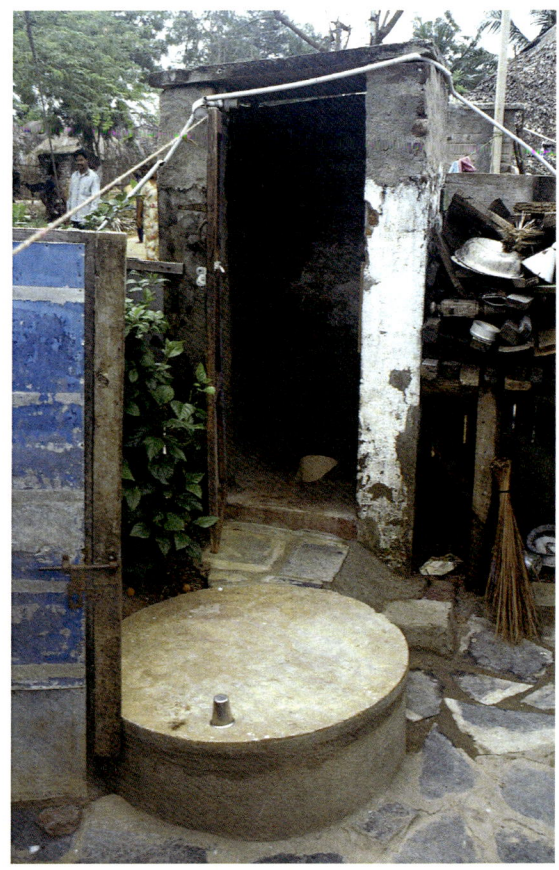

FIGURE 11 Urban and rural populations without access to improved sanitation in East Asia, 2008

The rural population without access to sanitation services in East Asia is almost half a billion people, which is over 60% more than the 300 million urban people that are not served.

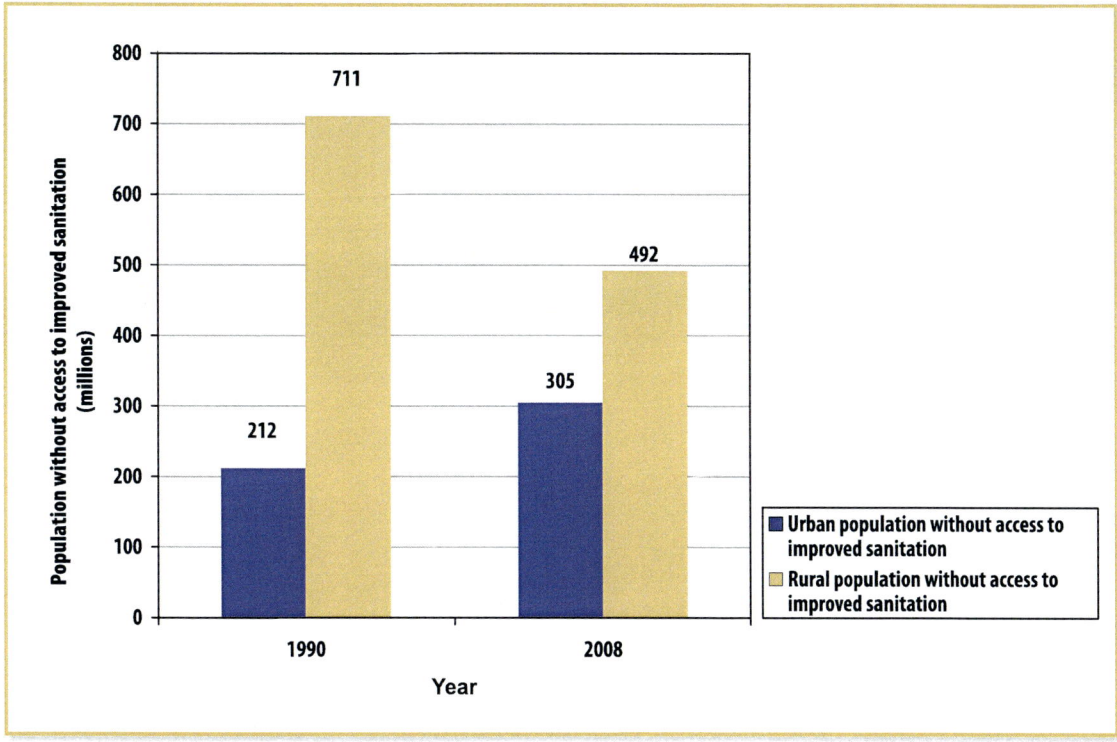

Source: Compiled from country coverage data from WHO and UNICEF JMP database

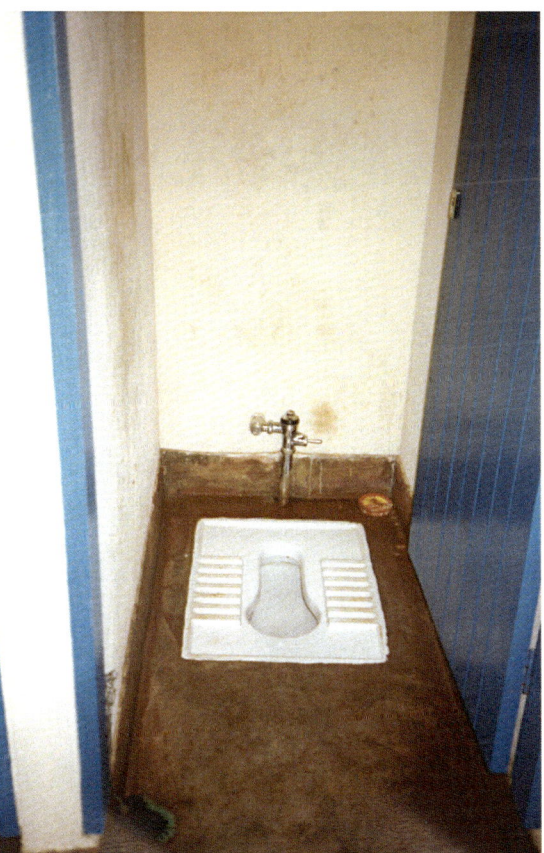

While the numbers of those not served with improved sanitation in East Asia decreased about 30% in rural areas, they increased over 40% in urban areas between 1990 and 2008. This is partly explained by the huge urban population growth, which exceeded 70% during the same period, while in rural areas the population remained practically constant over 18 years. Despite these changes, there remains a huge disparity in access to improved sanitation services in urban and rural areas (Figure 11).

Achieving the sanitation targets

Are the MDG sanitation targets achievable?

Most countries in East Asia for which information is available are either on track to achieve the MDG sanitation target or have already achieved it (Figure 12). Although this is an indication that the Region made good efforts to improve sanitation status, it is prudent to view these statistics realistically.

First, the Region as a whole is not on track to achieve the MDG sanitation target. It will fall short by 6 percentage points in 2015 of the MDG sanitation regional target of 74%.

Second, those achieving the target are the higher income countries such as Japan and Singapore, whose current national efforts went much beyond access to sanitation services because the large majority of their citizens enjoy access to fully regulated services. These countries are now focused on improving the quality of their sanitation services through massive investments in their wastewater treatment facilities and similar action to protect the environment.

Third, these statistics do not give an indication of the quality of the services provided. The numerous household surveys used by the JMP (Demographic and Health Survey (DHS), Multiple Indicator Cluster Survey (MICS), the

FIGURE 12 Proportion of people using improved sanitation in 2008, projected proportion of people using improved sanitation in 2015 and respective country MDG sanitation target in East Asian countries[1]

Although a half of the lower income nations in East Asia have already met the MDG sanitation target or are on track to achieve it, the Region as a whole will miss the target by six percentage points if the current coverage trend remains unchanged.

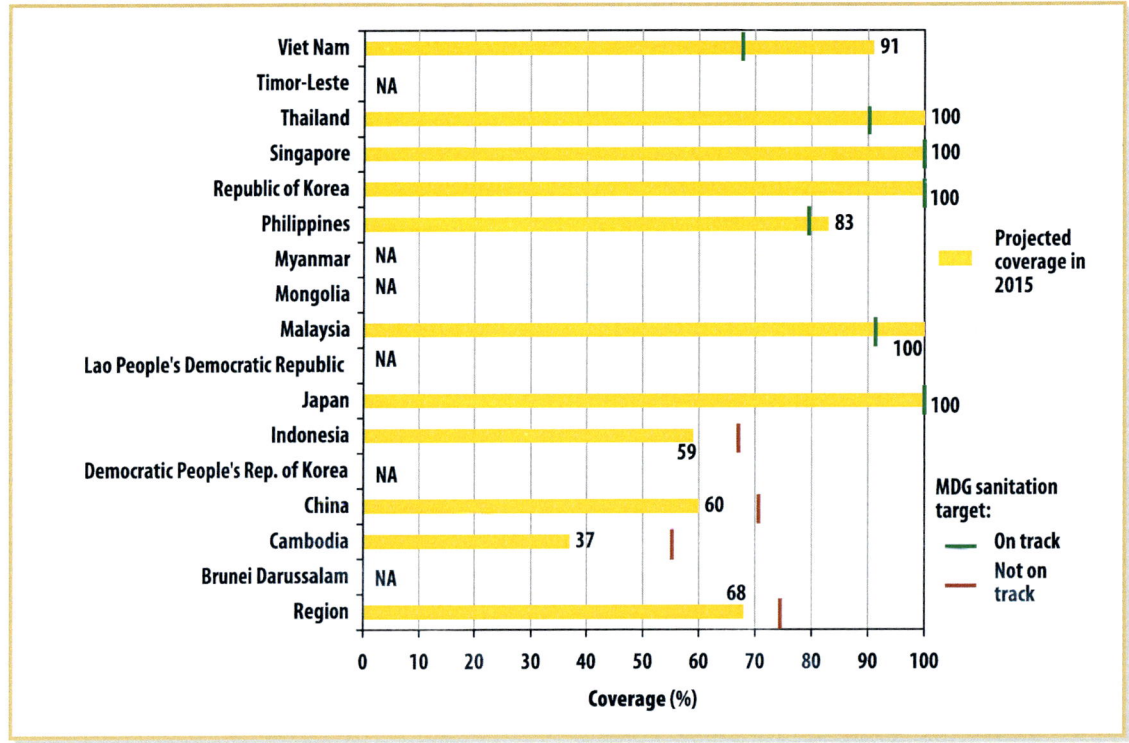

Source: Compiled from country coverage data from WHO and UNICEF JMP database

[1] Figure 12 provides the MDG targets and coverage projections calculated according to trends provided by the JMP statistics. They might differ from official national coverage statistics and targets.

World Health Surveys (WHS) and national censuses) to estimate sanitation coverage do not include an assessment of cleanliness and whether the sanitation facility effectively protects health.

Fourth, achieving the target does not mean necessarily an optimum level of services to those having access to improved facilities. It is likely that even if the targets are achieved, there will remain major challenges to harmonize people's needs with environmental and health requirements. Some of the "improved" sanitation technologies may be hazardous to both existing sources of drinking-water and the environment in the neighbourhood of the household. For example, public sewerage systems discharging untreated sewage into bodies of water may inflict serious harm to the environment downstream. The discharge of raw sewage into coastal areas may affect the food chain through fish and shellfish. Septic tanks with soak pits and latrines below the water table may contaminate precious groundwater sources.

There is an urgent need to conduct national surveys that take these factors into account for an effective determination of different levels of services and their relationship to health and the environment.

It is also important to emphasize that several countries for which a trend is not available (the Lao People's Democratic Republic, Mongolia, Myanmar and Timor-Leste) have low coverage and likely would increase the statistics of countries not achieving the MDG sanitation target if such a trend was available.

Despite the negative analysis above, there has been remarkable sanitation progress in East Asia since less than half of the population at the baseline year of 1990 used improved sanitation

FIGURE 13   Change in the proportion of people with improved sanitation between 1990 and 2008 and projection of change in East Asia between 2008 and 2015

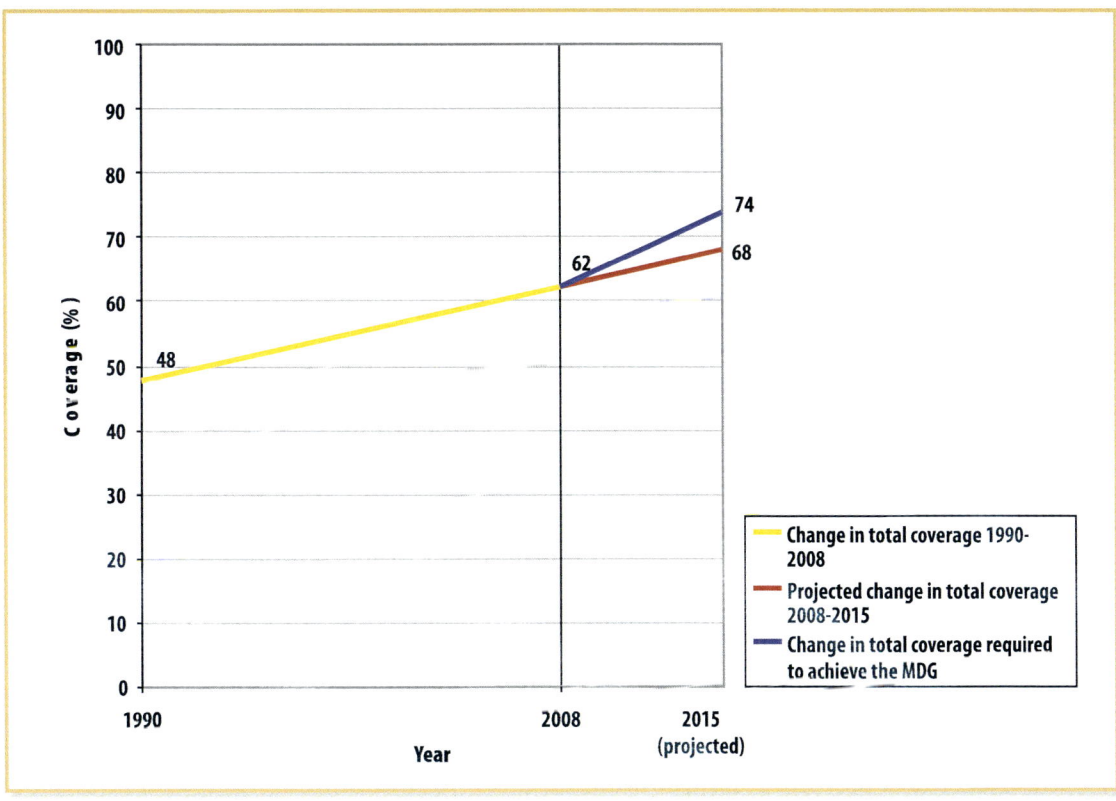

Source: Compiled from country coverage data from WHO and UNICEF JMP database

facilities (Figure 13). Increasing the coverage by 14 percentage points during a huge population growth is proof that much greater progress can be achieved should the East Asian countries accelerate investments to improving sanitation. Less encouraging is that about one-third of the population (about 700 million people) will remain without access to improved sanitation in 2015 (Figure 14). Even if the MDG sanitation target is achieved, over one-fourth of the East Asian population will not be served.

FIGURE 14 Change in population with improved and unimproved sanitation between 1990 and 2008 and projection of change between 2008 and 2015 in East Asia

Access to improved sanitation in 2015 will be almost double that of 1990 in East Asia, an impressive achievement. Despite this major effort, about one-third of the regional population still will not be served in 2015.

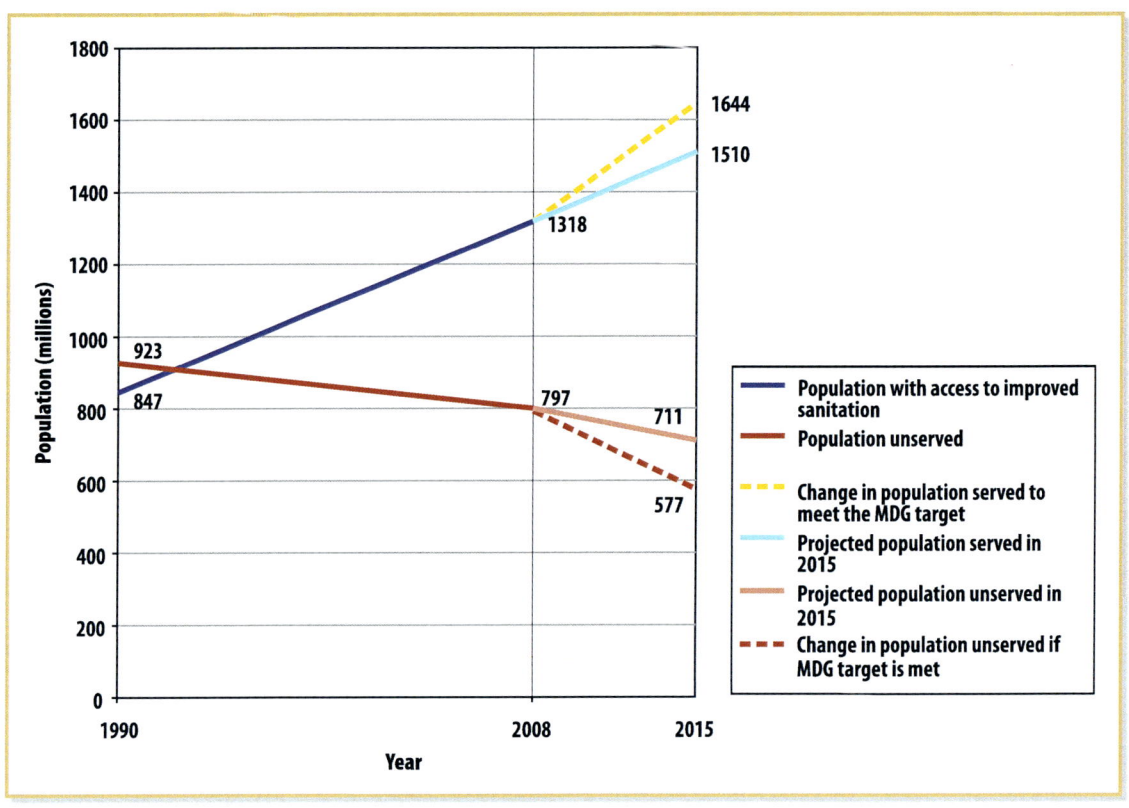

Source: Compiled from country coverage data from WHO and UNICEF JMP database

Monitoring sanitation

Comparing global and local coverage statistics

Global monitoring of access to sanitation provides unquestionable benefits in comparing country coverage status and in measuring progress towards international targets. However, globally-managed monitoring systems do not necessarily generate all the information needed to meet the country-specific requirements of information for policy-making and for planning and programming nationally and subnationally. At the same time that countries have specific needs and require tailored indicators to measure progress towards meeting such needs, it is likely that the resulting information might not be comparable with that produced by other countries or by the JMP. Where monitoring systems at the country level are based on evidence rather than on subjective assumptions, it is possible to reconcile and harmonize the information generated by these systems with those of the JMP.

How different are the JMP coverage statistics from the official national statistics?

The official urban and rural coverage statistics provided by East Asian countries to the TWG WHS template showed a relatively small deviation as compared to the statistics provided by the 2008 JMP coverage revision (Figures 15 and 16). China, Mongolia and Viet Nam

FIGURE 15   Proportion of people using improved urban sanitation in East Asian countries, according to official national statistics and the JMP, 2008

Only two East Asian countries reported official urban coverage statistics that differ more than 15 percentage points from the JMP 2008 statistics.

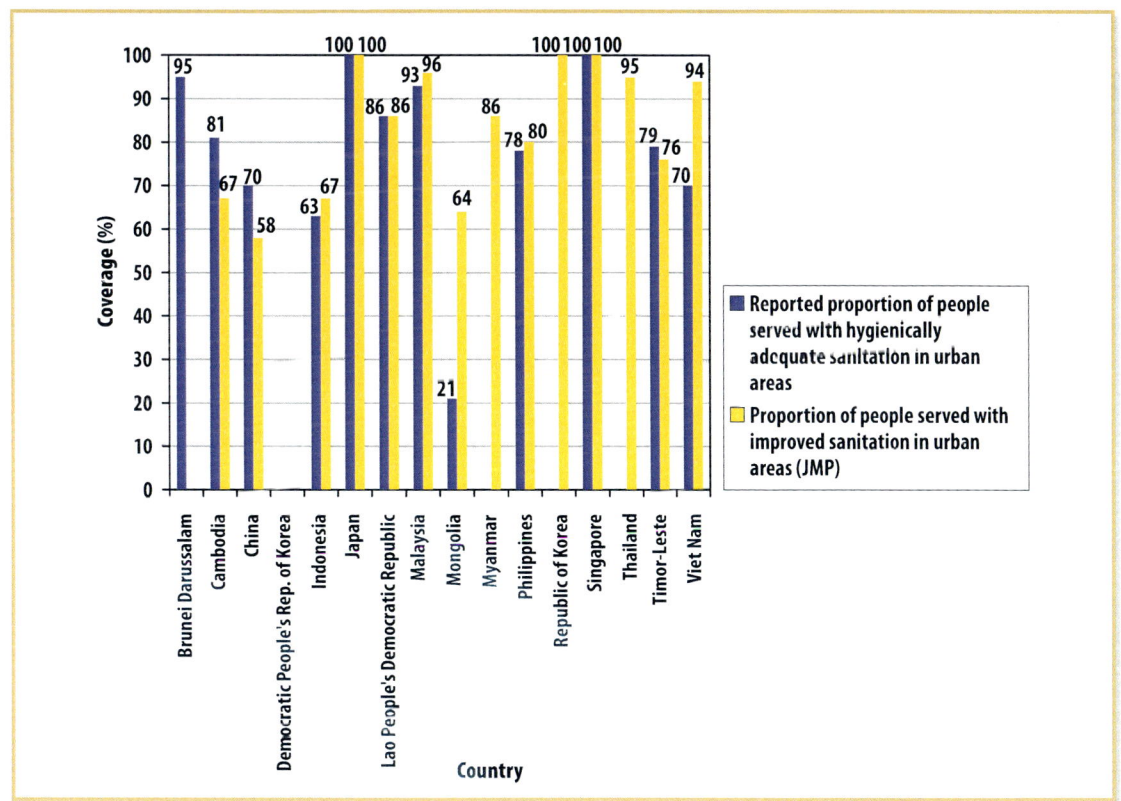

Source: WHO, UNICEF (2008) and primary data from country templates

FIGURE 16 Proportion of people using improved rural sanitation in East Asian countries, according to official national statistics and the JMP, 2008

Three Asian countries reported official rural coverage statistics that differ 15 percentage points or more from the JMP 2008 statistics.

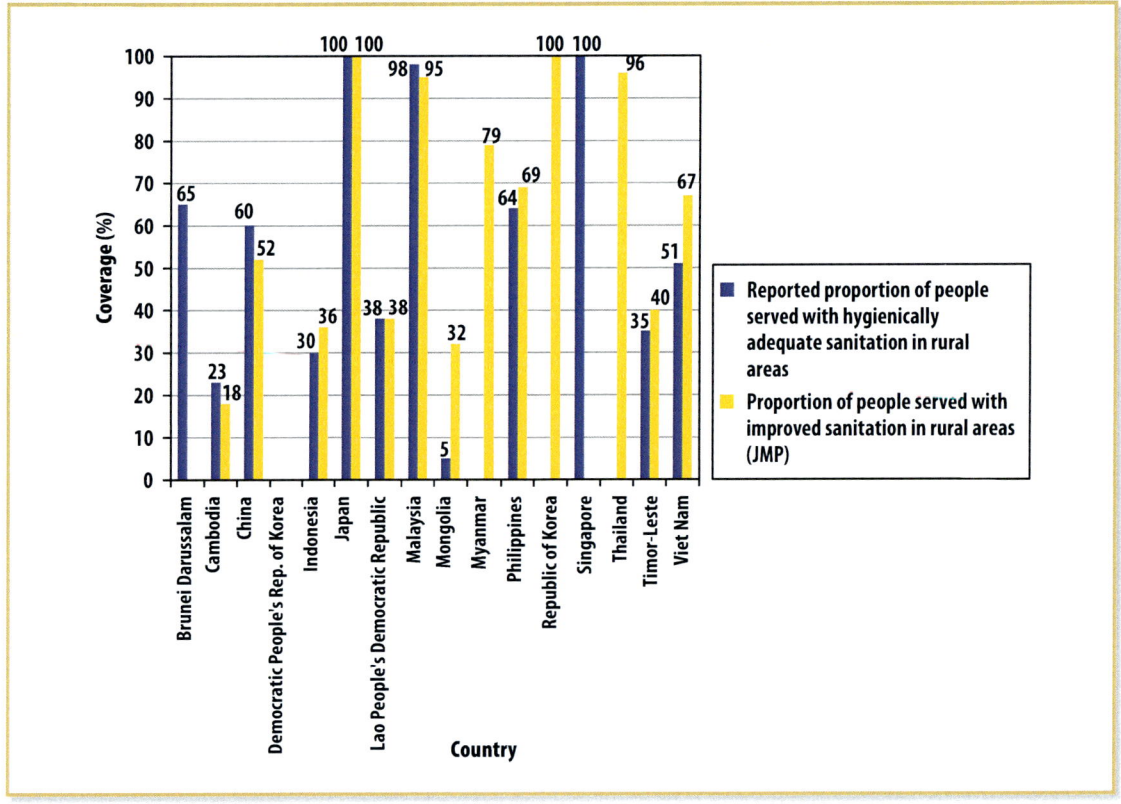

Source: WHO, UNICEF (2008) and primary data from country templates

present considerable differences because their definition of adequate access to sanitation differ considerably from the definition of improved sanitation by the JMP (Tables 1 and 3).

The differences between global statistics such as those produced by the JMP and nationally derived estimates as shown in Figures 15 and 16 may be because of a wide range of possibilities. For example, some countries may only consider as an acceptable type of access to sanitation services the availability of a toilet flushing to a sewerage system whereas the JMP considers various other types of sanitation facilities as improved. Some countries may consider sharing improved sanitation facilities as improved whereas the JMP considers them as not improved.

Discrepancies also may occur because of the method of measurement. While the JMP uses household surveys as the primary source of information to derive coverage statistics, some countries might adopt information given by the providers of services as the national standard. Even where household surveys are adopted as the source of information, the outputs of such surveys may be defined according to a method that may differ from that used by the JMP, which would probably generate disparity in coverage figures.

Other approaches often used by governments to derive sanitation coverage statistics, which differ from the JMP approach, include the following:

- Use of local governments and communities to determine access to services: a common approach (e.g. Viet Nam, the Philippines) is to collect information about every household through forms filled out by a local government office;
- Use of information about existing infrastructure to derive access to services; and
- Where the water services are managed by a water utility, the latter will use its users' registering system to derive the

population served. In many cases, the utility might have information about the users connected to their sewerage system but are unlikely to have reliable information about users of on-site sanitation.

What is considered acceptable in terms of access to sanitation?

As indicated in a previous section, different countries have different standards about what is acceptable and what is inadequate. While in the Republic of Korea and Singapore the standard

TABLE 2 Types of sanitation facilities considered hygienically adequate or inadequate by East Asian countries

	Types of sanitation facilities considered as hygienically adequate	Types of sanitation facilities considered as hygienically inadequate
Brunei Darussalam	• Centralized sewerage system • Septic tank system	• Wastewater discharged directly into water bodies (without treatment).
Cambodia	• Flush or pour-flush to sewerage • Flush or pour flush to septic tanks or pit • Pit latrine with slab • Ventilated improved pit latrine.	• Public or shared latrine (any type) • Flush or pour-flush to elsewhere • Open pit latrine without slab • Latrine overhanging water
China	**Urban:** • piped sewer system • septic tank **Rural:** • Pit latrine with slab • composting toilet	
Indonesia	• Water-flush-type Latrine • Gooseneck latrine • Pit latrine	• Bored-hole Latrine • Bucket Latrine • Trench Latrine • Overhung Privy
Japan	• Sewerage • Johkasou (private wastewater treatment system) • Waste collection and treatment system	No toilet

The Lao People's Democratic Republic	• Flush or pour-flush to:
	  - piped sewer system
	  - septic tank
	  - pit latrine
	• Ventilated improved pit latrine (VIP)
	• Pit latrine with slab
		• Pit latrine without slab or open pit
		• Bucket
		• Hanging toilet or hanging latrine
		• No facilities or bush or field (open defecation)
		• Public or shared sanitation facilities

Malaysia	• Flush toilets properly connected to sewer • Flush toilets connected to septic tanks • Sanitary pit privy • Other devices approved by the Department of Sanitation	• Open pit latrine • Over hung toilets
Mongolia	• Centralized public sewer system • Local sewerage systems/septic • Pour-flush latrine with seat • Ventilated, lined pit latrines • Lined, adequate soak pit	• Simple pit latrine • Open pit and screened hole • Bucket latrine • Unsealed soak pit
The Philippines	• Flush toilets properly connected to sewer • Flush toilets connected to septic tanks • Sanitary pit privy • Other devices approved by the Department of Health	• Open pit latrine • Over hung toilets
The Republic of Korea	Public sewerage	
Timor-Leste	• Pit latrines, flush toilets and septic tank as the means of final disposal of sewage. • Ventilated Improved pit latrine (VIP)	• Pit latrine without a easy to clean slab, a fly proof lid, a ventilation pipe with fly proof screen • Traditional latrine combined with pig-shed
Viet Nam	• Septic tank • Pour flush latrine • Double vaults latrine • Ventilated improved pit latrine.	• Fish pond connected latrine • Pit latrine • One vault latrine

Source: TWG WHS country templates

sanitation option is toilets flushing to a well-regulated sewerage system, other countries adopt the concept of improved technologies similar to those of the JMP. Table 3 shows the types of sanitation facilities considered as hygienically adequate or inadequate in selected East Asian countries.

Is there a suitable system for monitoring sanitation coverage?

Five countries (China, Indonesia, the Philippines, Timor-Leste and Viet Nam) reported that they have national monitoring systems that are not well coordinated, resulting in conflicting information from different agencies. Three countries (Cambodia, the Lao People's Democratic Republic and Mongolia) indicated that they have sound monitoring systems but they are not well integrated into review and planning. Brunei Darussalam and the Republic of Korea indicated that they have a sound monitoring system, well-coordinated, with a clear definition of responsibilities, which is integrated into sector review and planning. None of the respondents reported having an ineffective monitoring system.

Crucial issues and important recommendations to improve national sector monitoring

Establishing a sound national monitoring system for hygiene, sanitation and water supply is an essential requirement to measure progress towards national targets and for identification of priority areas of intervention. Having a well-coordinated national and subnational monitoring system capable of measuring both the availability of sanitation facilities, including the types of such facilities, their state of maintenance and cleanliness, their use by all members of the household and the practise of good hygiene, should be essential elements of sound national monitoring.

Although the above monitoring elements are crucial for a definition of priorities, policy-making, planning and allocation of resources, there is a need for more information to provide for a more complete understanding of the sector status. For example, more is needed to be known about national institutional frameworks, roles and responsibilities, operation and maintenance

---

BOX 2 National water supply and sanitation sector assessments

The WHO Western Pacific Regional Office and UNICEF East Asia and Pacific Regional Office are promoting and supporting national water supply and sanitation sector assessment programmes aimed at collecting and analysing information and producing recurrent evidence-based reports on the performance of the national drinking-water and sanitation sector.

The specific objectives of such national programmes are:

- To demonstrate the relationship of drinking-water, sanitation and hygiene to health and economic growth as an evidence-based instrument to stimulate informed strategic decisions at the country level;
- To support continuing national planning and policy reform initiatives;
- To guide technical assistance programmes; and
- To serve as a platform to accommodate exchanges of information through an Internet-based database collected for the sector analysis.

A document titled "Establishing a Drinking-Water and Sanitation Sector Assessment Process: A Guide for Country-level Action" has been recently published by WHO and UNICEF to help broaden the implementation of sector assessment programmes in the Region. National assessment programmes are under way in the Philippines and Viet Nam with support from WHO, UNICEF and the United States of America Agency for International Development (USAID).

Source: WHO/WPRO, UNICEF/EAPRO (2009)

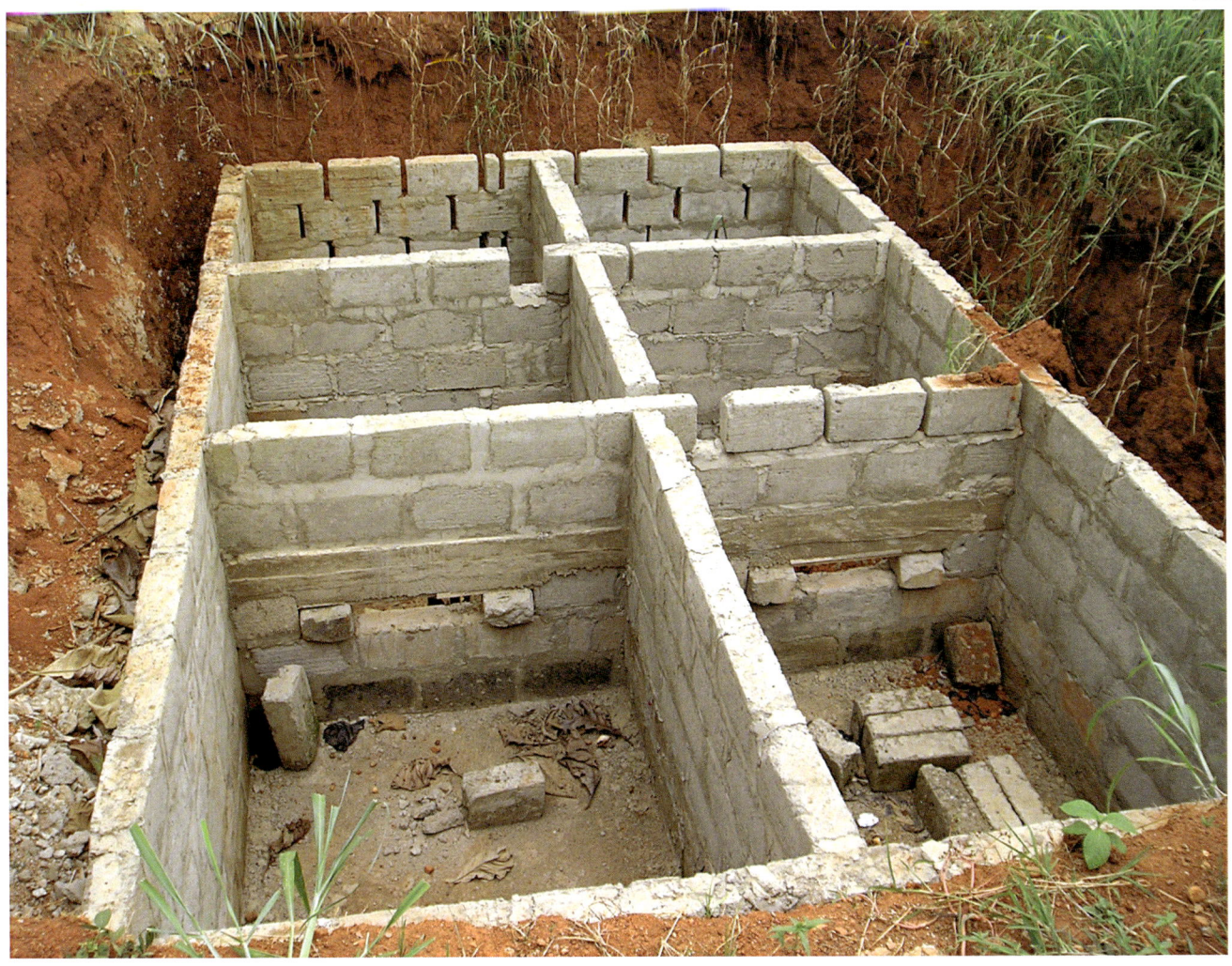

practises, finance and a good deal of other information for a better understanding of the sector performance as a whole. Box 2 summarizes a water and sanitation sector assessment initiative led by the WHO Western Pacific Regional Office and UNICEF East Asia and Pacific Regional Office, which is under way in the Philippines and Viet Nam before it is broadened to include the whole Region.

According to the East Asian respondents to the TWG WHS templates, the following factors are, in summary, essential to improve monitoring in their countries:

- Establish a national comprehensive monitoring system with a standardized definition of indicators, proper definition of responsibilities, good coordination and collaboration mechanisms and a well-formulated methodology to generate and use information;
- Establish a national monitoring committee for hygiene, sanitation and water supply with the primary function of unifying and coordinating monitoring at the national level;
- Define the financial mechanisms to ensure the sustainability of the monitoring system;
- Assign adequate monitoring staff at central and sub-national levels;
- Establish a consolidated national database for water, sanitation and hygiene unifying monitoring systems from various agencies; and
- Encourage participatory monitoring.

Why is hygiene so important?

The combination of poverty, poor health and lack of hygiene means that children from homes without sanitation facilities miss school more frequently than those whose families benefit from improved drinking-water and sanitation services. The resulting lack of education and social development further marginalizes the children and reduces their future chances of self-improvement. It is well known that three priority water-related hygiene behaviours have a greater impact on the incidence of diarrhoeal diseases: hand washing, sanitary disposal of faeces and keeping drinking-water free from faecal contamination. Fewtrell L et al. (2005) estimated that improved sanitation and good hygiene behaviour reduce diarrhoeal diseases morbidity by an average of 32% and 45%, respectively.

Effectiveness of hygiene education programmes

Figure 17 provides a summary of the answers to the question: "How effective are the hygiene education programmes in your country"? The lack of indicators to substantiate the responses weakens the analysis since it is based merely on the perception of the respondents. Despite such a drawback, it is obvious that hygiene education programmes in the region require improvement.

In response to the question whether there is a national hygiene and sanitation strategy or plan, five countries (Brunei Darussalam, the Democratic Republic of Korea, Indonesia, Japan and Viet Nam) reported that they have a comprehensive strategy or plan in place for which there is full government support and that they are widely put into effect. Five countries (Cambodia, China, the Lao People's Democratic Republic, Mongolia and Timor-Leste) indicated the existence of a partial strategy or plan to which limited support is provided and is not fully in effect.

All of the countries reported that their national programme for hygiene promotion include components such as social mobilization, communication, social marketing, community

FIGURE 17 Perception of the effectiveness of hygiene education programmes in selected East Asian countries

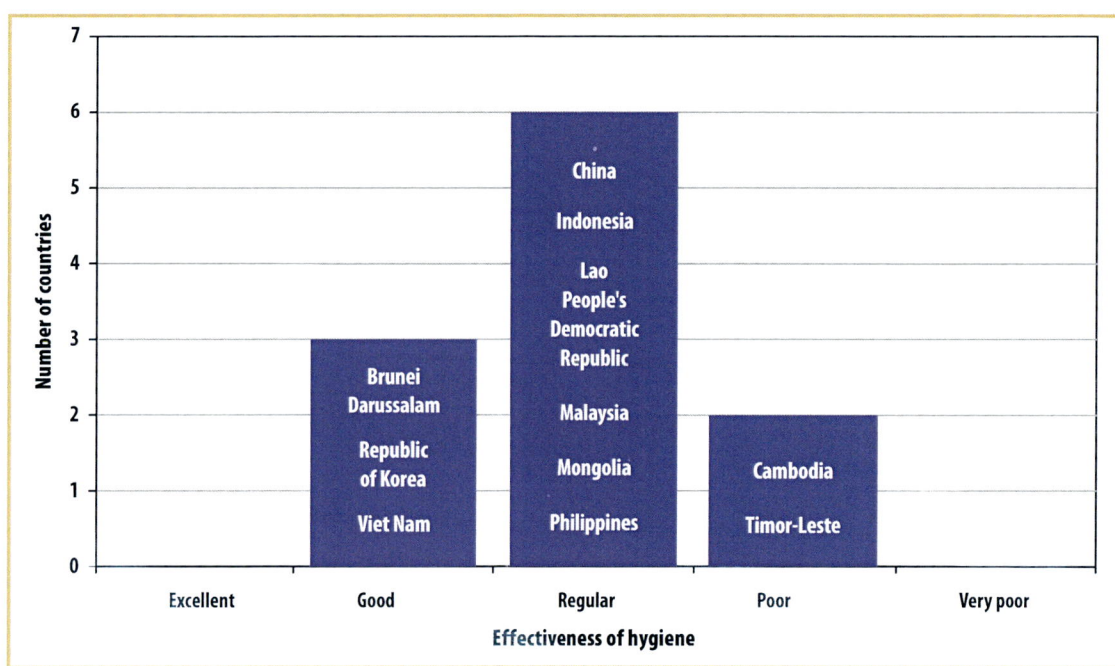

Source: TWG WHS country templates

participation and advocacy. For example, in Cambodia, Hygiene and Sanitation Transformation (PHAST) is the approach adopted to promote hygienic practices in rural areas. In Mongolia, hygiene promotion is included as an important element of both the Health Master Plan and the Sanitation Programme approved by the Mongolian Government in 2005 and 2006, respectively. The hygiene promotion sections of these documents include communication, social marketing and advocacy for communities and professionals. In Indonesia, the National Strategy for Community-Based Total Sanitation includes five pillars: stop open defecation, wash hands with soap, household drinking-water and food management, household solid waste management and household wastewater management. For all pillars, activities involving social mobilization, communication, social marketing, community participation and advocacy are undertaken to put the national strategy into effect widely. In Timor-Leste, the national programme for hygiene promotion, organized by Ministry of Health, through Integrated Community Health Services, includes behavioural change communication and demonstration of good hygiene behaviours.

Hygiene behaviour in primary schools

Brunei Darussalam, the Lao People's Democratic Republic, the Republic of Korea, the Philippines, Timor-Leste and Viet Nam reported that hygiene behaviour is included effectively in the primary or secondary school curricula in their countries as opposed to Cambodia, China, Indonesia and Mongolia, where this is not carried out effectively.

Key issues to improve hygiene

The hygiene problems, constraints and recommendations identified by the East Asian countries include the following:

Constraints and problems:

- Lack of a synchronized approach and strategy at national and subnational levels;
- Lack of financial support for hygiene promotion;
- Discontinued support from donors because sanitation and hygiene promotion interventions require a long time to produce sustainable results;
- Low level of education of people in rural areas;
- Poverty;
- Inadequate water and sanitation systems in rural and remote areas;
- Many ethnic groups in remote areas need targeted materials on information, education and communication;
- Difficulty in changing the education levels, attitude and behaviour of rural people, especially those in remote areas.
- Lack of information and weak behavioural change communication system.

Recommendations:

- Create awareness among policy-makers of the importance of hygiene promotion;
- Formulate a national hygiene promotion plan to improve the levels of hygiene at all levels with proper budgets and a clear definition of roles and responsibilities;
- Revise existing primary and secondary school curricula so they include hygiene promotion effectively;
- Improve the effectiveness and reliability of hygiene monitoring and evaluation;
- Increase the frequency of communication for hygiene education using the different media nationwide;
- Organize training at the local level to promote and facilitate social mobilization and community participation for improvement of hygiene behaviour;
- Actively involve the local government and communities in hygiene promotion programmes;
- Support from stakeholders at all levels needs to be increased for better regulation, policies and financial support; and
- The provision of sanitation services must be community-based to ensure their sustainability.

Investing in sanitation and hygiene

Discussion of this chapter should centre on whether the levels of investment in sanitation and hygiene promotion in Member States increase over time and whether a special focus on sanitation occurs on its own or if it occurs to the detriment of investments in the water supply. An assessment also should be made about whether the planned investment in sanitation is likely to lead to the achievement of the MDG sanitation target and other national targets.

Unfortunately, little information has been provided through the EASAN2 template, which was insufficient to establish trends and provide a reliable analysis. This means there is an acute lack of information about national investments in sanitation. This is true either because these investments are so irrelevant that they are not worth measuring or because there is a lack of reliable information systems capable of generating this information.

Worldwide, according to WHO (2008) (Hutton and Bartram), lower income countries worldwide must spend US$ 142 billion between 2005 and 2015 to provide new coverage to meet the MDG sanitation target. The cost of maintaining existing services totals an additional US$ 216 billion for sanitation. Additional programme costs of between 10% and 30% are required for effective implementation. Unfortunately, there is no specific rigorous economic analysis for the group of countries included in this analysis. This important issue should be included as a crucial one in the cooperative agenda for EASAN2.

Annualized investment spending on sanitation

As indicated above, it is a daunting task to obtain investment information about sanitation at national level. There are several reasons for this acute lack of financial information. First, most countries do not have a centralized information system about sanitation and water that would make it easily available. Second, the sector is normally highly fragmented and there is little coordination among the different players that otherwise would allow information to flow in an organized and effective manner. Third, the investments and recurrent expenditures in sanitation and water supply are frequently bundled and it is difficult, if at all possible, to produce a breakdown of these figures. Fourth, the investments made at the household level are normally not captured by national statistics mechanisms. It has been demonstrated that a lack of access to improved sanitation services seriously can harm the economic growth of a nation (Box 3).

Major initiatives, plans or programmes

Table 4 summarizes the information reported by selected TWG WHS Member States on their respective sanitation initiatives. This list is not intended to be exhaustive. It provides a hint of country-level action, which represents the greatest impact to improving sanitation, in the view of the respondents.

What is being done to increase demand for sanitation services by households and consumers?

The low level of demand for sanitary means of excreta disposal has been recognized as a major cause of failure of sanitation programmes. It is well known that the main motivation for the user's investment in sanitation facilities is definitely not health, as was believed until recently. Other reasons take priority, such as reducing odours and flies, privacy and pride in the cleanliness of areas surrounding the household. Thus, it is crucial to have a clear understanding of this motivation and use the right communication strategy to stimulate demand. Marketing sanitation and promoting behaviour change are key areas that still need to be emphasized and supported since merely a few countries have encouraged extensively the required skills,

BOX 3 Economic impact of sanitation in South-East Asia

A study conducted recently involving Cambodia, Indonesia, the Philippines and Viet Nam (Hutton G et al, 2008) revealed that these countries lose an estimated US$ 9 billion a year because of poor sanitation (based on 2005 prices) and that this is about 2% of their combined gross domestic product (GDP) (1.3% in the Philippines and Viet Nam, 2.3% in Indonesia and 7.2% in Cambodia). Indonesia has the highest economic losses, either in total or as a value per capita.

Universal sanitation would lead to an annual gain of US$ 6.3 billion in the four countries. Poor sanitation has a potentially negative impact on several aspects of a nation's economy. The study focuses on five areas because of their importance or amenability to analysis using credible information and data sources: health, water resources, environmental (focusing on the outdoors), other welfare (focusing on preferences for latrine type) and tourism. The study found that health care costs because of a lack of adequate sanitation produce the highest economic losses as compared with other categories.

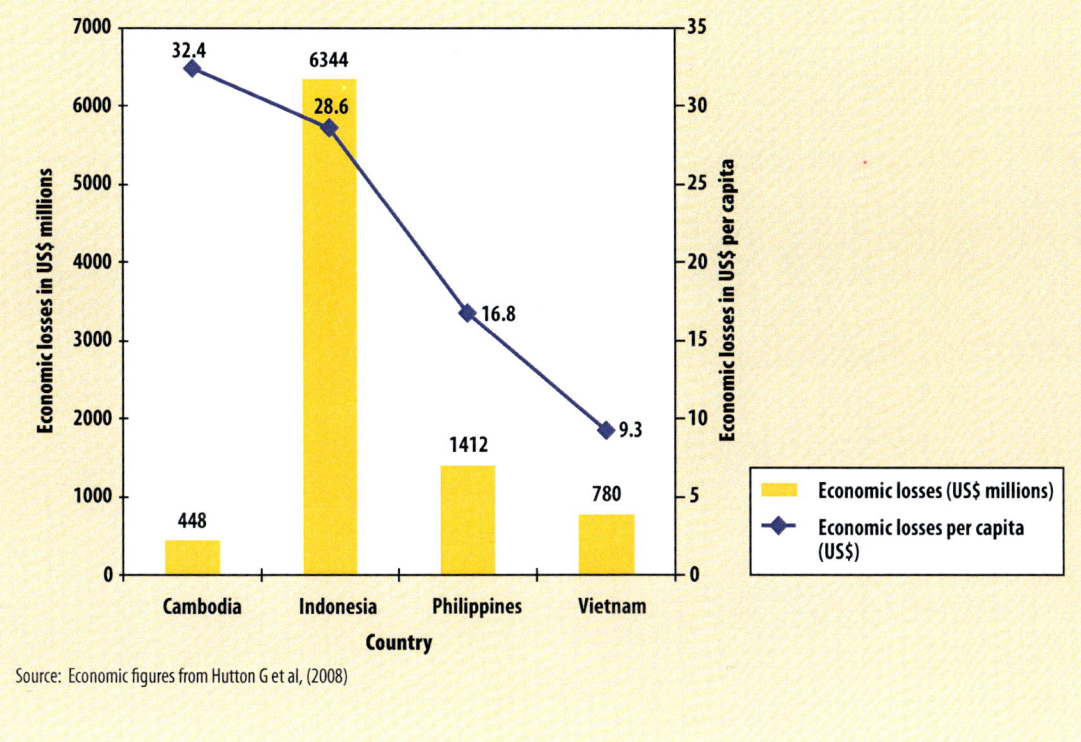

Source: Economic figures from Hutton G et al, (2008)

incentives and capacities to undertake effectively such important areas. This is a priority area in the reshaping of public sanitation programmes (Evans, B, 2004).

Regional countries asked what is being done to increase demand for sanitation services by households and consumers gave the following responses:

- In Brunei Darussalam, the households using on-site septic tanks are offered a free connection to the existing sewerage system.
- In Cambodia, there is a programme to generate sanitation demand in rural areas through social marketing.
- In China, the demand for sanitation services is being generated through an increase of financial resources and strengthening of policies. One policy calls for a hygienic sanitation facility in each newly built household.
- In Mongolia, training and awareness are being transmitted to communities through both official and unofficial media channels.

TABLE 3 Initiatives, plans or programmes on sanitation as reported by East Asian countries

Country	Initiative, plan or programme	Objectives/targets
Cambodia	Accelerated and sustained progress on sanitation and hygiene assisted by the United Kingdom Department for International Development (DFID) and UNICEF; low-cost latrine promotion programme assisted by WSP and International Development Enterprises Cambodia (IDE-Cambodia).	Not provided.
China	National Hygiene and Sanitation "Eleventh Five-Year Plan", which is the national plan for hygiene and sanitation.	Increase sanitation coverage in rural areas to 65% by 2010; by 2010, the proportion of public toilets in municipalities and provincial capital cities will not be less than 70%.
Indonesia	The National Strategy for Community-Based Total Sanitation (CBTS).	Its aim and objective is to be used for reference in planning, implementing, monitoring and evaluating the community-based total sanitation program.
Mongolia	National Environmental Health programme by Mongolian Government in 2005 aimed at building a healthy environment for living and working. This will be achieved by action on risk factors linked to the contamination of the environment as well as through an improvement of intersectoral collaboration.	Between 2006 and 2010: Strengthen monitoring and legal systems; enhance evaluation of adverse health impact; implement actions on reducing morbidity related to environmental pollution; promote sustainable ecosystems; and improve health education.
	United Nations Joint Programme on Water and Sanitation in Mongolia. The goal of this UNDP, UNICEF, WHO and United Nations Population Fund (UNFPA) programme is to increase water and sanitation provision at local levels by improving water and sanitation management.	Between 2009 and 2011: Strengthen legal and regulatory frameworks; improve knowledge and behaviour change; enhance national database, taking into account the JMP methodology; improve capacity of drinking-water quality monitoring; increase water and sanitation provision at local levels; improve community ownership over water sources and sanitation facilities.
	National Programme for Sanitation Facilities aimed at improving sanitation facilities at all levels and constructing or maintaining sewerage treatment plants.	First phase between 2006 and 2010; Second phase between 2010 and 2015.
The Philippines	Preparation of the Sanitation Roadmap.	Duration: between August 2009 and January 2010. Document will serve as a guide for the sanitation subsector. Will define priority strategies, outcomes and outputs for the next medium-term development plan.
	Preparation of the National Sewerage and Septage Management Plan.	Duration: between June and November 2009. The document is the national strategy for large-scale sanitation interventions addressing sanitation and sewerage in highly urbanized areas.
The Republic of Korea	To implement sewerage maintenance project by watershed.	To improve water quality of watershed regions while enhancing efficiency in budget execution through building and operating comprehensive sewerage projects based on watershed regions.
	To put into effect a project for maintenance of sewerage systems in rural villages.	Active investment is necessary to increase the sewerage connection rate of marginalized rural areas while managing existing facilities handed over from the Ministry of Public Administration and Security
	The government invested the equivalent of US$ 30 billion between 1992 and 2008 in building sewerage infrastructure and connecting users to the respective systems.	The sewerage connection rate increased from 39% in 1992 to 89% in 2008.
Viet Nam	National Target Programme for Rural Water Supply and Sanitation funded by the government and donors Danish International Development Agency (DANIDA), the Australian Agency for International Development (AusAID) and the Netherlands Directorate-General of Development Cooperation (DGIS). This programme focuses on intersectoral cooperation, information, educational and communication (IEC) activities, research, capacity building and technical assistance and pilot sanitation models such as ecological sanitation, latrines for flood areas and social marketing of sanitation. It encourages rural households to build hygienic latrines by themselves.	By 2010: • 85% of rural households will have access to clean water • 70% of rural households will have access to a hygienic latrine; • 100% rural kindergartens, primary schools and commune health clinics will have clean water and hygienic latrines.

Source: TWG WHS country templates

- In the Philippines, social marketing of sanitation is under implementation by civil society organizations and concessionaires of sanitation services. A Community-Led Total Sanitation (CLTS) programme is under way in pilot areas under the leadership of the Department of Health. A similar approach has been adopted in Timor Leste.
- In Viet Nam, there is an extensive programme on communication, information and education for changing behaviour and building latrines.

Stakeholders participation

This section of the report briefly assesses the level of participation and involvement of different sanitation stakeholders such as women, children, poor families, civil society and the public and private sectors in the planning and implementation of sanitation and hygiene programmes.

The assumption that people defecate in the open because they cannot afford a toilet or that a subsidy will boost demand for a toilet have been found to be erroneous (Mukalla, R, 2008). Community-driven total sanitation approaches appear to work more effectively in poor areas than the traditional approach focused on subsidies for household and public toilets and grants for urban sewerage and solid waste systems. Traditionally, the approach to providing access to sanitation has been supply-driven and focused on financing the building of toilets, installing sewerage networks and constructing treatment facilities. A review of emerging thinking and practise suggests that a shift in sanitation financing is required from financing "subsidies and grants for sanitation facilities" to funding "sanitation promotion and leveraging resources" (WSP/Africa, 2004).

Encouraging local governments to pay attention to sanitation

Decentralization of sanitation and water supply management has been promoted across East Asia extensively. In many countries, this approach was not followed up by support for local-level planning, definition of priorities, identification of financial mechanisms to upgrade the sector and capacity-building. Consequently, the level of effort towards sanitation improvement at the local government level is less than adequate in various countries.

Very few respondents to the TWG WHS questionnaire reported effective action to stimulate local governments to play a more active role in sanitation improvement. A few responses included the following:

- The national government in China supports local governments' action on sanitation through funds and policies formulation. It has been a strong advocate of reforms in rural areas with the active participation of local governments to expand access to basic sanitation and water supply services and to create replicable models for expanding such services.
- In Indonesia, activities including socialization, advocacy and training (capacity-building) are conducted by the central government to the provincial, district and city governments for widespread implementation of CBTS programmes.
- In the Philippines, the national government supports local governments through awareness-raising, capacity-building and access to financing.
- In Viet Nam, the central government exerts efforts to strengthen local governments through information and capacity-building and supports their consolidation as the responsible administrative level for sanitation promotion and implementation.

Participation of women, children, poor families and the public and private sectors in planning and implementing sanitation programmes

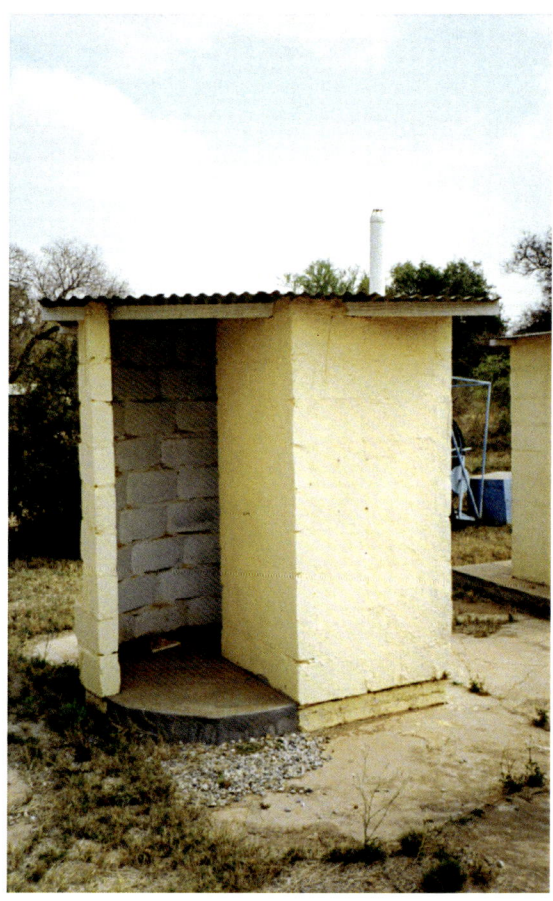

The East Asia countries were asked through the TWG WHS template whether the participation of women, children, poor families and the public and private sectors in planning and implementing sanitation programmes was excellent, sufficient or insufficient. Only two countries responded that it was sufficient (the Lao People's Democratic Republic and Republic of Korea). All of the others indicated that such participation was insufficient.

According to Cairncross S (2004), evidence from what works in lower income countries indicates that marketing sanitation is a sustainable approach to meet the need for sanitation in poor areas. His suggested method of marketing sanitation consists, in synthesis, of the following steps:

- **Win consensus:** Establish a policy consensus on adopting this approach, including a policy on subsidies. This may be difficult at the national level, especially where the government follows a centralized approach and is the main provider of services. Implementation could start at a subnational level. It is crucial to identify a champion at the local level to lead the process and influence others to adopt it.
- **Learn about the market (demand and supply):** On the demand side, learn what people do to meet their sanitation needs, who helps them, at what expense and why. On the supply side, there is a need to learn more about existing latrine builders, pit emptiers and other sanitation service providers, which can yield valuable insights into their sales, costs and prices and constraints to increased demand and increased production.
- **Overcome barriers, promote demand:** Make existing regulation more supportive, for example, by removing restrictive building regulations and replacing them with manuals on how to build various models of low-cost sanitation facilities. Advertising campaigns can be organized nationally whereas production and sales are best organized locally.
- **Create the right products:** Although the market system is fundamental to the success of a sanitation programme, there is also a need to create adequate products. Families have different needs and require product choices that meet those needs.
- **Create a booming industry:** Stimulate creation of the local private market in view of the greater demand to be expected from demand promotion, especially to meet the needs of the poor.
- **Regulate waste transport and final disposal:** Public subsidy and regulation of the disposal of wastes outside the home should be established, taking into account that most low-cost latrine types are on-site systems requiring regular emptying and safe disposal.

BOX 4   A Cambodian village decides to bring sanitation closer to home

Villagers in Slaeng, 60 km southwest of Phnom Penh, made a crucial commitment in rural Cambodia. They decided to abandon open defecation, an ancestral practice, and to use proper sanitation facilities. Over three years, every single household built a toilet, and the 452 inhabitants resolved to use them. This huge behavioural change is extraordinary, considering that until recently people thought it deeply distasteful, even frightening, to squat over the dark pit of a household latrine.

What is the secret behind the Slaeng villagers' abandonment of the bush and adoption of a closed toilet instead? The answer is twofold. Local leadership, from Mr Chan, the chief, and others he enlisted, and an approach by the authorities that focused on encouragement and motivation, not imposition of an idea from outside.

A striking feature of the approach was the absence of external financial or material subsidies. Past projects offered subsidies of US$ 25 as an incentive to construct sanitation facilities, but most of the households that accepted such subsidies were not the poor or in need of it. No one later copied their example and adopted toilets voluntarily, so the impact was negligible among the poorest and least healthy families. What made a big difference in this project was the participation of the villagers in discussing the problem and analysing the solutions themselves.

The approach to community-led total sanitation now being applied in Cambodia was pioneered in Bangladesh and is being replicated in countries all over Asia and Africa. This is an innovative way of mobilizing communities to eliminate open defecation through active participation and community analysis and action without the use of subsidies for every household to build their own facility.

Source: UNICEF (2009)

BOX 5 Why people want latrines

A survey of rural households in the Philippines elicited the following reasons for satisfaction with a new latrine. The reasons are listed in order of importance, starting with the most important:

- lack of flies;
- cleaner surroundings;
- privacy;
- less embarrassment when friends visit; and
- reduced gastrointestinal disease.

Although health is an important motivator to behaviour change and to eliciting efforts from householders to have sanitary latrines at home, it appears that other motivators such as dignity, convenience and social status are viewed as having even a higher priority by the users. A major finding of this study is that sanitation promotion should be based on arguments that are closer to the heart of the potential users than that of policy- and decision-makers and sanitation promoters.

Source: Adapted from WHO, UNICEF (2000)

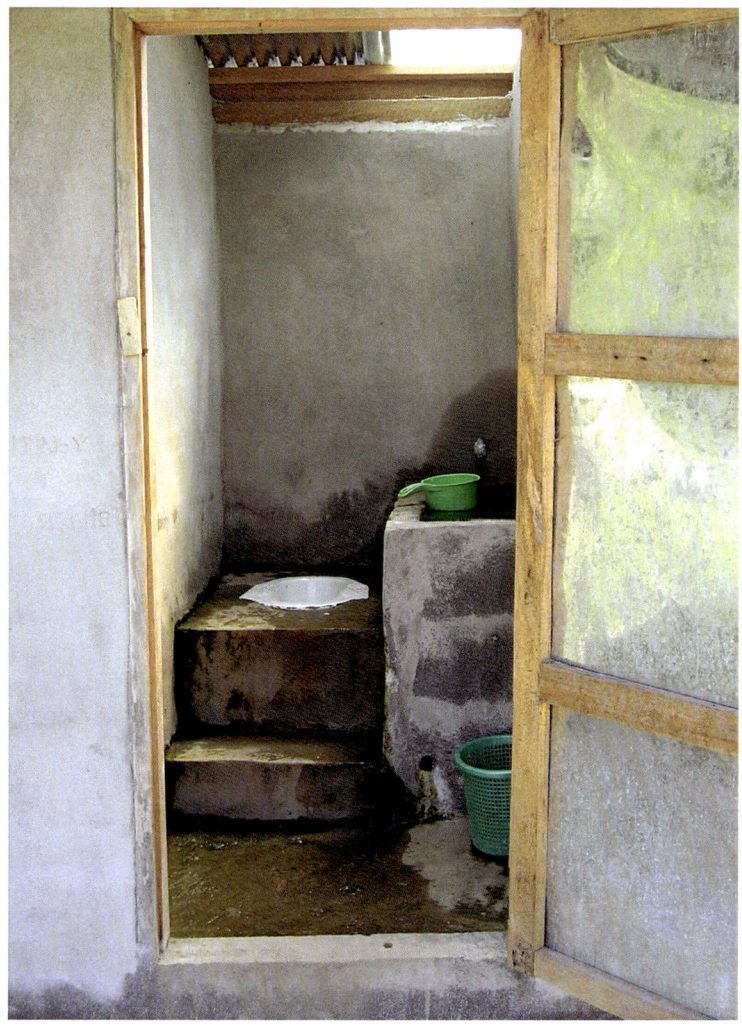

What is being done to stimulate private sector participation?

It is largely recognized that the private sector has a crucial role to play in sanitation development, from the most remote rural communities to large urban sewerage systems with costly and complex wastewater treatment plants. The modalities of such participation need to be defined according to local legislation, institutional framework, financial aspects, local culture and political considerations. It can vary from simple contracts for basic maintenance services to the overall management of a utility, including the ownership of assets.

The East Asian countries were asked about actions to stimulate private sector participation. There are a number of successful experiences in the Region. Some of them are summarized as follows:

- In Cambodia, a manual for household latrine selection was prepared and disseminated to Government agencies, NGOs and local private sector. Awareness raising activities (modelled on CLTS approaches) stimulate demand for the latrines, and efforts to link to local micro credit providers are in an advanced stage. There is a waiting list of suppliers wanting to be trained in the approach. Cambodia also has embarked on a School-Led Total Sanitation Programme which relies extensively on the supply of materials and services by small entrepreneurs.
- In Indonesia, the socialization and implementation of CBTS programmes requires extensive use of local private entrepreneurs.
- In Mongolia, under the framework of the Soum Hospital Project funded by WHO, the sanitation facilities of 20 soum hospitals were constructed or maintained through contracts awarded to private entrepreneurs.
- In the Philippines, the Metropolitan Waterworks and Sewerage System functions under successful concession contracts which permit steady improvement of the Metro Manila sanitation system. Public-private partnerships are encouraged at local levels. A successful example is the decentralized wastewater treatment facilities operated privately in partnership with local governments.
- In the Republic of Korea, legal frameworks are being formulated and guidelines are being formulated to establish concessions for private companies for the management of wastewater treatment facilities.
- In Timor-Leste, individual entrepreneurs are being encouraged towards sanitation component production and sale under a pilot sanitation marketing initiative in one district.
- In Viet Nam, private companies are being encouraged to establish latrine construction services. Also, commune mason groups are being stimulated to build latrines in direct connection with households.

Sanitation and hygiene in schools and health care facilities

This section of the report looks into the status of sanitation facilities and hygiene practices in schools and health care establishments. It assesses whether sanitation facilities in such establishments are adequate and provide the means for practising hygienic behaviour. An assessment is made of the proportion of schools and hospitals and health care centres that have adequate sanitation facilities and whether there are plans to improve the status of such services.

Proportion of public primary and secondary schools with adequate sanitation facilities

The country responses to the TWG WHS templates indicate that the information available on the status of sanitation in public primary or secondary schools is remarkably weak. There is usually no monitoring system in place to measure the availability and quality of sanitation services in these facilities. Figure 18 shows the statistics presented by a few countries where reported information is available.

FIGURE 18   Percentage of public schools having adequate sanitation facilities in selected East Asian countries

The proportion of public schools with adequate sanitation facilities presented in this graph hints a cruel reality: there are many public schools devoid of basic sanitation facilities. The consequence is that children, most of them girls, are deprived of primary or secondary education because they cannot live with the embarrassment of having no access to decent hygienic sanitation facilities while attending classes.

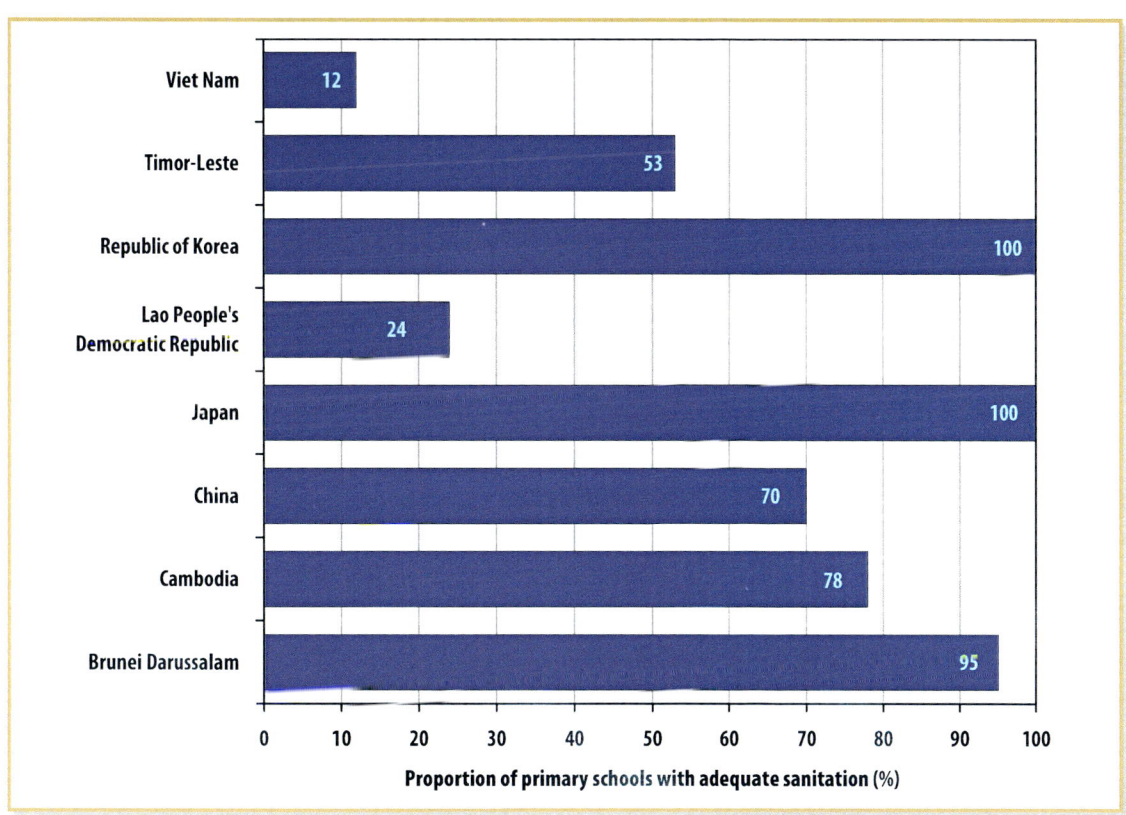

Proportion of primary schools with adequate sanitation (%)

Source: TWG WHS country templates

In Cambodia, China and the Philippines, water supply and sanitation facilities originally were built in most public schools. But the lack of operation and maintenance made most of them unusable or put them in such a state of disrepair that they no longer encourage use. Mongolia and Viet Nam believe that both the quantity of sanitation facilities in each school and their quality should be improved substantively. They also believe that such facilities are not managed properly after their construction.

In Mongolia, the quality of sanitation in schools is acceptable in cities where sewerage systems are available. But it is very poor in rural areas, namely in most soum centres, villages and in peri-urban areas. In these zones, unimproved pit latrines and soak pits are the standard. They are often unlined and there is no privacy or safety for children. In addition, hand-washing basins are not available for the majority of the sanitation facilities in most soum centres. In Timor-Leste most schools do not have functional toilets and hand washing facilities.

Proportion of public hospitals and health care centres with adequate sanitation facilities

Public hospitals and health centres should have sanitation facilities and hygiene orientation that should serve as a model for other settings. However, reality shows a much different scenario. First, it was obvious from the responses to the country templates that there is little information available about this issue. Second,

FIGURE 19   Proportion of public hospitals and health care centres with adequate sanitation facilities in selected East Asian Countries

With only 37% of the public hospitals and other health care centres with adequate sanitation facilities in Viet Nam, 30% in Mongolia and 80% in China, it is strongly probable that nosocomial infections are rampant in most of these establishments.

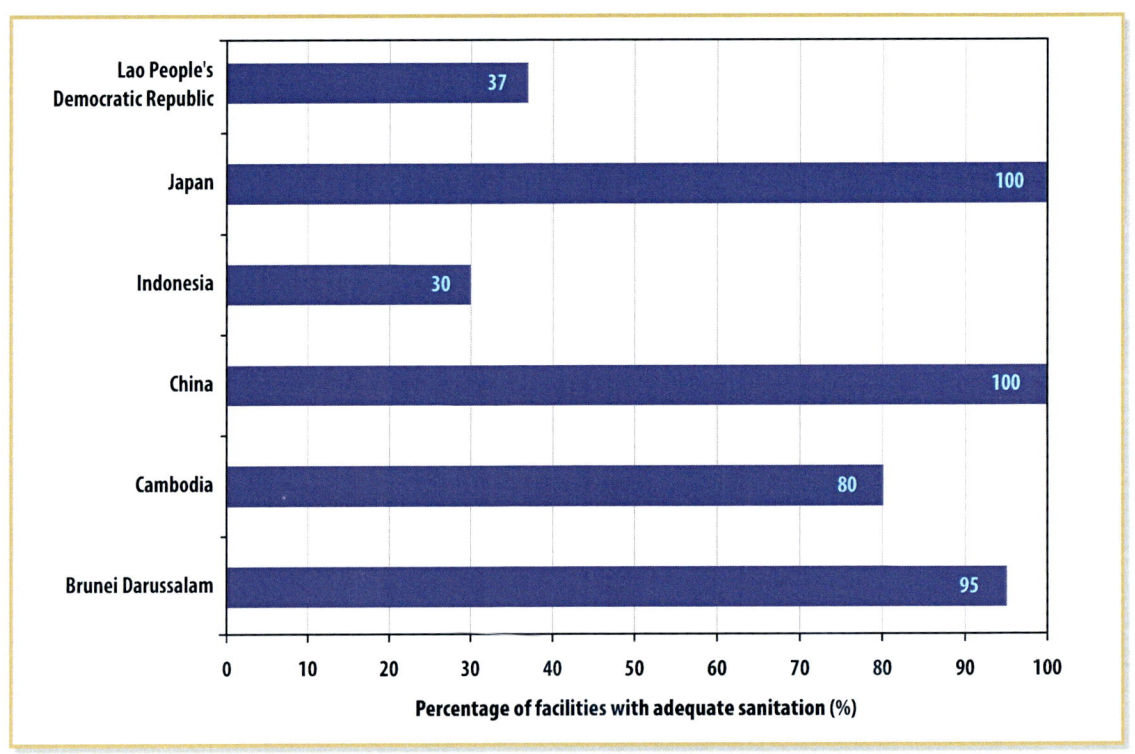

Source: TWG WHS country templates

the information available indicates a reality that is distant from acceptable (Figure 19).

Most TWG WHS countries reported major problems related to insufficiency of sanitation facilities and their precarious state of disrepair, filth and poor maintenance. In addition, there is no system to monitor systematically the state of sanitation and hygiene in public health establishments. Therefore, there is little evidence-based information available for promotion and advocacy.

What should be done to improve the level of sanitation services in schools and health care establishments

Table 4 provides the views of the TWG WHS countries on how to improve sanitation in schools and health care facilities.

TABLE 4   Recommendations for the improvement of sanitation and hygiene in public schools and health establishments in East Asian countries

Area	Recommendation	Countries recommending
Promotion, policies and strategies	Promote and encourage the active participation of students in the proper operation and effective maintenance of sanitation facilities.	Cambodia
	Increase the commitment of local governments.	Indonesia
	Increase awareness about hygiene and healthy life behaviour.	Indonesia
Legal framework	There is a need for formulation and approval of a sound regulatory framework for schools and health care establishments dealing with sanitation and drinking-water requirements.	China
Institutional framework	Intersectoral cooperation needs to be strengthened for a better definition of responsibilities and effective action.	The Lao People's Democratic Republic Mongolia
Financing	The government should realistically allocate financial resources for construction and operation and maintenance of public schools and health care establishments in national financial planning.	China The Philippines Viet Nam
	Build in operation and maintenance costs in management of the sanitation facilities. Ensure the availability of the water supply.	The Philippines
	School principal or head of health care establishment needs to be active in fund-raising for operation and maintenance within the community served by these establishments.	Cambodia The Lao People's Democratic Republic
Monitoring and evaluation	Monitor regularly levels of service and progress jointly by the education ministry and the local health authorities.	The Philippines Timor-Leste
Human resources	Strengthen local human capacity to improve the level of operation and maintenance of sanitation facilities.	Mongolia

Source: TWG WHS templates

How are institutions organized to face the sanitation challenge

The sanitation and hygiene institutional framework

The responses to the TWG WHS templates indicate that the responsibilities for sanitation, especially rural sanitation, are not clearly defined and are an afterthought in different national or local agencies. The responsibilities for sanitation and the communication and coordination mechanisms among agencies appear to be blurred in most countries and in some cases simply do not exist (Figure 20).

FIGURE 20 Governmental responsibility for sanitation in East Asian countries

The responsibility for sanitation in East Asian countries ranges from a situation in which no coordination is attempted (Cambodia) to a situation where the responsibilities for sanitation are well defined, well understood, with inter-departmental coordination working effectively (Japan).

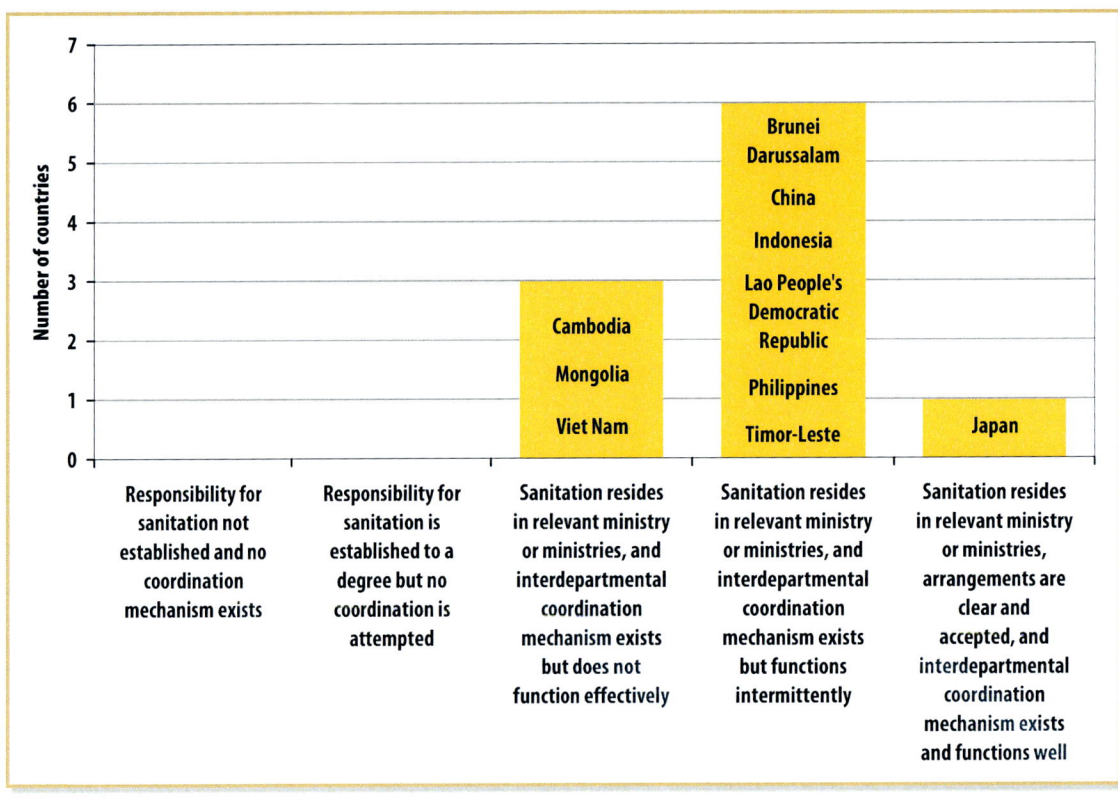

Source: TWG WHS templates

The countries responding the TWG WHS templates also were asked for their views about how to improve the organization of the sector and the national institutional framework for sanitation. Table 5 summarizes the TWG WHS template responses accordingly.

Key issues to take into account to improve human resources

For any sanitation structure to function effectively, there is a need for well-trained personnel with professional and personal credentials compatible with the requirements of the respective posts. There is a need to characterize correctly the required profiles of the different sanitation posts and to meet them accordingly with existing or new personnel. There is also a need to create incentives, through adequate salaries and an effective career-building plan, to attract and keep qualified professionals, adequate staff productivity levels for service providers and analyse if sector and national personnel policies in the country recognize the need for any adjustment.

Figure 21 indicates in general terms the perception of the respondents to the TWG WHS template on

TABLE 5 Recommendations and issues on the sanitation and hygiene institutional framework in East Asian countries

Countries recommending	Recommendation
Brunei Darussalam Mongolia Timor-Leste Viet Nam	There is a need to establish a clear institutional framework for sanitation, including the definition of roles and responsibilities of different national and subnational stakeholders.
The Lao People's Democratic Republic The Philippines Viet Nam Cambodia Mongolia	Sanitation and hygiene responsibilities cut across many agencies. Thus, interagency and intersectoral coordination mechanisms should be effectively established.
The Philippines	There is a need for a strong sanitation sector champion and the establishment of a national technical assistance mechanism for local implementers.
Cambodia China	There is a need for resource mobilization (financial, human resources) for implementation of rural sanitation strategies and programmes.
The Lao People's Democratic Republic	There should be a decisive local political commitment to sanitation improvement and more financial and technical support from international agencies to country-level sanitation improvement.
China	There should be more emphasis on human resources training, especially at the management level.

Source: TWG WHS templates

the level of training and sufficiency of different types of sanitation staff across the region.

Figure 21 indicates that while there is an overall international stimulus to decentralize sanitation services towards local governments and communities and involving the local private sector to move forward the sanitation agenda, the personnel in these settings is simply not properly trained in sufficient numbers to assume such an important and difficult responsibility. How to resolve this crucial issue? The TWG WHS templates contain relevant information on this crucial issue, as shown in Table 6.

FIGURE 21 Level of training and sufficiency of sanitation personnel in East Asia

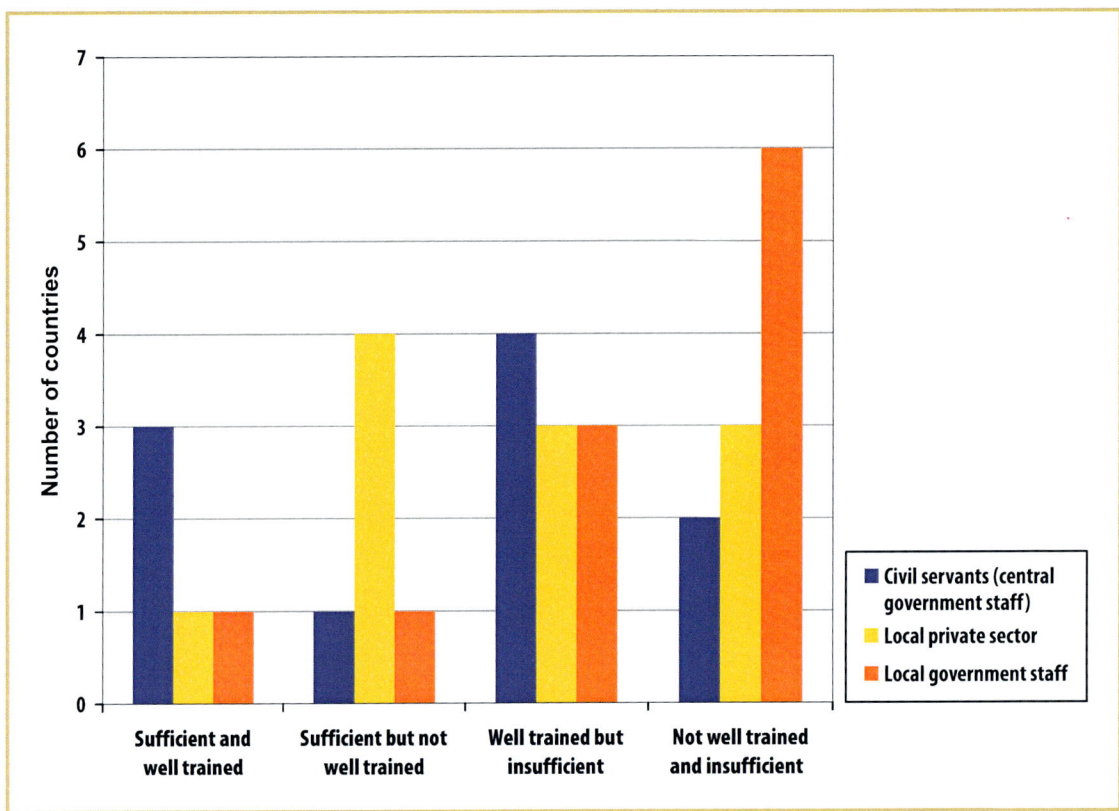

Although most sanitation personnel are not well-trained, this is especially true among local government staff and the local private sector.

Source: TWG WHS country templates

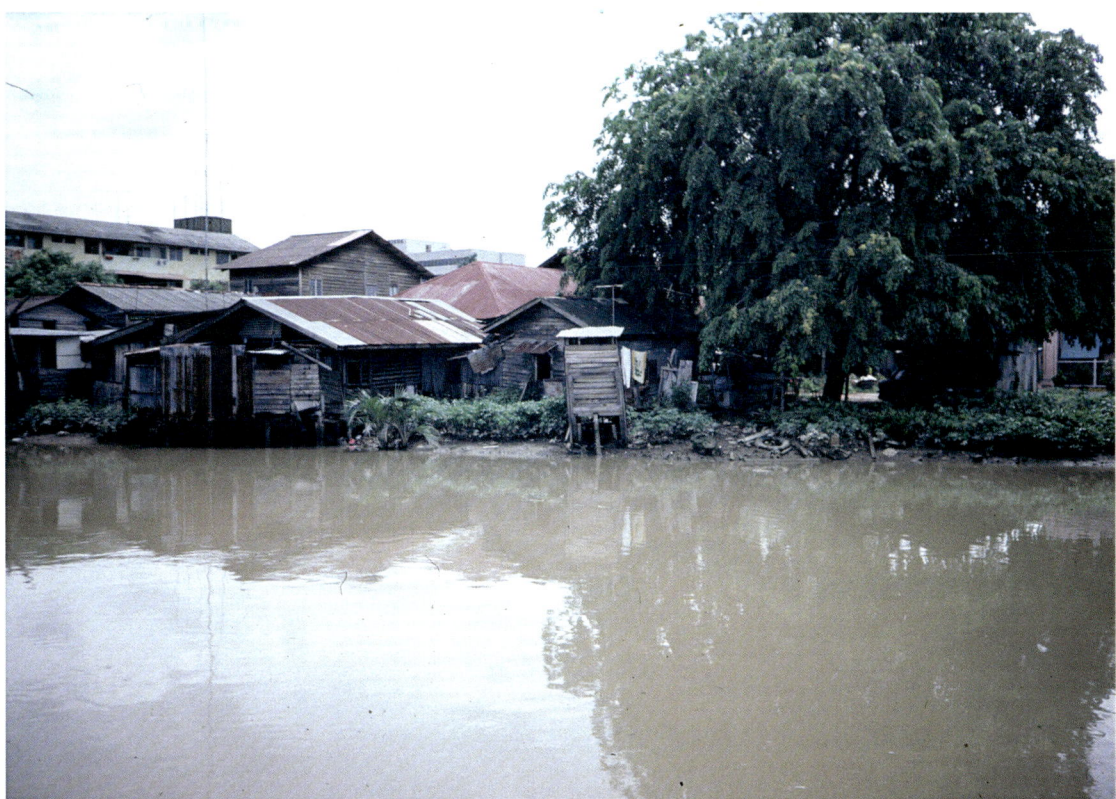

TABLE 6 Recommendations for sanitation and hygiene human resources improvement in East Asian countries

Countries recommending	Recommendation
Cambodia Indonesia The Lao People's Democratic Republic Mongolia Viet Nam The Philippines Timor-Leste	Allocation of financial resources for capacity development, including the establishment of training facilities and postgraduate short-term training at the country level and abroad. Increase the numbers and quality of sanitation and hygiene staff at the subnational level (districts, provinces, villages).
Brunei Darussalam China The Republic of Korea	Emphasize the training of managers and technical staff in sanitation and hygiene and formulate strategies to keep high-quality sanitation and hygiene personnel.
Cambodia	Devise incentive mechanisms to avoid the turnover of effective sanitation and hygiene staff at all levels, but especially at the local authoritative level.
	Formulate and implement clear and feasible strategies on human resources training.
China	Put into effect a sanitation and hygiene qualification authentication system for technical staff and gradually expand the qualification requirements of such staff accordingly.
Indonesia The Lao People's Democratic Republic Viet Nam	Continuous training and sharing of experiences among villages; improve information, education and communication materials; more international cooperation for education exchange.
Mongolia	Create incentives for professionals working in remote areas through the improvement of their living conditions and increase of salaries.
The Philippines	Professionalize sanitation inspectors within the state career development process.
	Stimulate demand for sanitation courses offered by indigenous training institutions and stimulate sanitation agencies to recruit personnel trained in such recognized institutions.
The Republic of Korea	To prepare a professional education course on sewerage so as to share know-how and information regarding the operation and management of advanced sewerage facilities; shift the educational focus from institution and theory to field and on-the-spot learning.

Source: TWG WHS templates

Why is this all happening

Perceived constraints for sanitation and hygiene improvement

The problem of sanitation has been discussed extensively over the last decades. Invariably, the main constraints hampering the improvement of sanitation and hygiene are recognized internationally as being the following:

- Lack of political will to recognize sanitation as a priority issue;
- Low importance given to sanitation as compared to other growth priorities;

TABLE 7 Constraints for sanitation improvement as perceived by East Asian countries

Area	Constraint	Countries indicating the constraint
Policies and strategies	Lack of a sound sanitation sector strategy; Lack of a policy on subsidies for the sanitation sector; Different subsidies provided by different nongovernmental organizations (NGOs).	Cambodia The Lao People's Democratic Republic Timor-Leste
	Sanitation is not a priority: no comprehensive policy and weak implementation.	The Philippines
	Difficulty to promote and support community participation, especially in remote areas; There is a lack of good guidelines for sanitation improvement.	Indonesia The Lao People's Democratic Republic
Legal framework	Inadequate regulatory standards.	The Philippines
Institutional framework	Lack of coordination among sector agencies, which hampers sanitation interventions, especially in rural areas.	Cambodia
	Weak and fragmented institutions; no lead agency.	The Philippines
	Little importance given to sanitation by local governments.	Brunei Darussalam Indonesia Viet Nam
	Poor operation and maintenance.	Brunei Darussalam The Lao People's Democratic Republic China Indonesia Mongolia The Republic of Korea
Financing	Lack of sufficient financial resources and financial mechanisms to ensure the construction of infrastructure, operation and maintenance and social marketing.	Cambodia China Indonesia The Republic of Korea Timor-Leste Viet Nam
Monitoring and evaluation	Inadequate monitoring and evaluation.	The Lao People's Democratic Republic Timor-Leste
Human resources	Lack of human capacity, mostly at provincial and district levels.	Cambodia Mongolia The Philippines Timor-Leste
	Lack of sound human resources within the private sector	Brunei Darussalam

Source: TWG WHS templates

- Inadequate or nonexistent policies on sanitation;
- Fragmented institutional framework;
- Overlapping responsibilities and gaps in sanitation management;
- Inadequate and poorly used human and financial resources;
- Inadequate approaches and inappropriate technologies;
- Low importance given to users' preferences;
- Poor promotion and low awareness at all levels;
- Poor operation and maintenance; and
- Children and women frequently are not a priority.

The request to the TWG WHS countries of grouping their perceived constraints to sanitation improvement in six major areas provided useful returns, which are summarized in Table 7.

The countries also were requested to rank these constraints for sanitation improvement. The top constraint identified by each country is shown in Table 8.

What can be done to solve the problem

How to solve the sanitation problem?

There is no universal answer. Different countries have different needs and different definitions of sustainable access to hygienic sanitation. However, it is universally accepted that solving the sanitation problem would require the achievement of universal coverage with sanitation systems that ensure effective health protection and are sustainable, not only in terms of continuity of services but also in preventing environmental pollution and ecological degradation. Solving the problem means also that the approaches and technologies used should be according to the different cultural and behavioural characteristics of the users. They should be affordable and compatible with the capacity of the users and managers to operate and maintain the systems. Finally, solving the problem should aim at universal coverage as a means to reduce inequity and as a critical condition to ensure dignity and opportunities of social and economic growth for all.

TABLE 8 Top constraints for sanitation improvement as perceived by East Asian countries

Country	Top constraint
Brunei Darussalam	Lack of sufficiently skilled and experienced consultants and contractors.
Cambodia	Lack of coordination mechanisms to harmonize rural sanitation development.
China The Lao People's Democratic Republic	Poor operation and maintenance.
Indonesia	Lack of community awareness on hygiene and sanitation behaviour (lack of education).
Mongolia Viet Nam	Insufficient financial resources for construction and operation of sanitation facilities.
The Philippines Timor-Leste	Sanitation is not a priority: no comprehensive policy and weak implementation.

Source: TWG WHS templates

BOX 6 Approaches to improve sanitation

A few different yet complementary approaches to improve sanitation have been put into effect successfully in poor areas of several countries as follows:

- Sanitation within a Sector-Wide Approach (SWAp) is applied countrywide. Scaling up uses government administrative and fiduciary systems. SWAps for water and sanitation are being used in Uganda and Tamil Nadu (in India);
- National sanitation programmes are being established in Bangladesh and India through total sanitation campaigns. These are community-led and use a people- centred approach with local governments and NGOs or, as in Lesotho, with limited subsidies and private sector involvement; and
- Citywide improvement for basic sanitation is practised in Ouagadougou, Burkina Faso, through sanitation promotion funded through a local sanitation surcharge. In Pune, India, community toilets are funded through the local authority's own resources and managed by communities and NGOs.

Source: WSP (2004)

BOX 7 The resilience of sanitation systems to climate change

Climate change may affect the availability of the water supply, which in turn affects the performance of water-borne sanitation facilities. This occurs either where the water supply is an important element of the technology process (e.g. flushing toilets) or where the capacity of the environment to absorb or reduce the adverse effects of wastewater is changed.

Where precipitation levels decline, sewerage systems may require an increased performance requirement, especially with regard to the wastewater treatment process, which will require more costly equipment and more effective operation and maintenance. This in turn will increase the cost and potentially the carbon footprint of wastewater treatment. While conventional sewerage systems, widely perceived as the gold standard sanitation technology, are only resilient to climate change in some scenarios, modified sewerage (e.g. condominial sewerage) is indeed more resilient to climate change.

On-site sanitation such as improved pit latrines and low-flush septic systems are more resilient to climate change than conventional sewerage systems. Pit latrines are resilient because different designs allow adaptation to changing climate. Some individual facilities may not be resilient. Where groundwater levels rise, pollution from pit latrines may become more difficult to control.

All sanitation technologies are vulnerable to climate change and all have some adaptive capacity. There is enough evidence to arrive at a general idea of which technologies are more and less likely to be resilient to climate change in a given region. But there is a lack of good tools to assess the climate change resilience of a technology in a given specific location. Creating such tools is a priority.

Adapted from WHO, DFID (2009)

> **BOX 8** Use of treated excreta and urine in agriculture
>
> The WHO guidelines for the safe use of wastewater, excreta and greywater (WHO, 2006) formulated specific recommendations for storage treatment of dry excreta and faecal sludge before use at the household level. The storage time is determined mainly by the ambient temperature. For temperatures between 2o and 20° C, a storage time of 1.5-2 years will eliminate bacterial pathogens (although regrowth of E. coli and Salmonella will need to be considered if rewetted) and will reduce viruses and parasitic protozoa below risk levels, although some soil-borne ova may persist in low numbers. Similar achievements will occur after one year of storage time for ambient temperatures from 20o-35° C.
>
> These guidelines also indicate that for all types of treated excreta, a recommended withholding time of one month between application of the treated excreta as a fertilizer and the time of crop harvest is required to reduce to acceptable levels the probability of infection.
>
> The recommended storage time for urine mixture (urine or urine and water) for both food and fodder crops that are to be processed is at least six months for the elimination of viruses and protozoa.
>
> For the use of urine as a fertilizer, there is a recommended withholding time of one month between application and crop harvest.
>
> Source: WHO (2006)

Is universal sanitation coverage a pipe dream?

There are major challenges to be tackled if universal sanitation is to be achieved in this Region. First, there is a need to keep pace with a rapid urbanization process underway in several countries. Most countries had an urban population growth ranging from 40% - 50% between 1990 and 2008. While the Region was predominantly rural in 1990, it will become predominantly urban in 2015. This means that adequate approaches and suitable technologies will need to be chosen as opposed to top-down approaches that proved to be ineffective in the past years.

Second, there should be more investments in rural sanitation, not only because it lags behind urban water supply and sanitation in many countries but also because health care is fragile in rural areas, making children and other vulnerable groups more susceptible to sanitation-related diseases.

Third, there should be improvement in the quality of sanitation services, and the sustainability of such services in urban and rural areas should be ensured.

Finally, it is crucial that suitable and reliable monitoring systems be in place not only to measure access (or lack of access) to sanitation services but also to measure the overall conditions and trends of the sector as a whole.

There has been a remarkable reduction in the proportion of people without access to improved sanitation facilities between 1990 and 2008. The proportion of people not served in 2008 was reduced to over 80% of the 1990 figures for both urban and rural populations (Figure 22) despite a huge population growth and a considerable migration of people from rural to urban areas.

FIGURE 22   Proportion of population in East Asia without access to improved sanitation facilities, 1990, 2008

Should the current coverage trend continue in East Asia, universal coverage will not be achieved in rural areas for another 40 years. It will be achieved in urban areas 90 years from now.

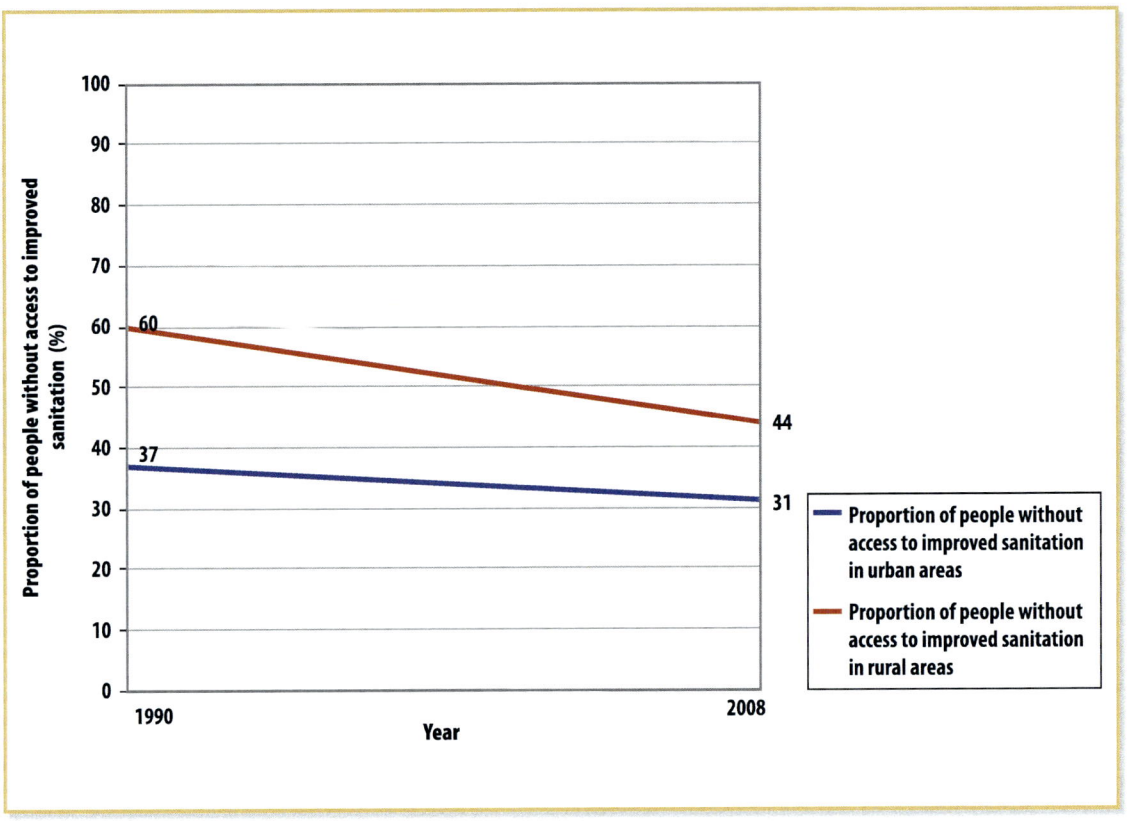

Source: Compiled from country coverage data from WHO and UNICEF JMP database

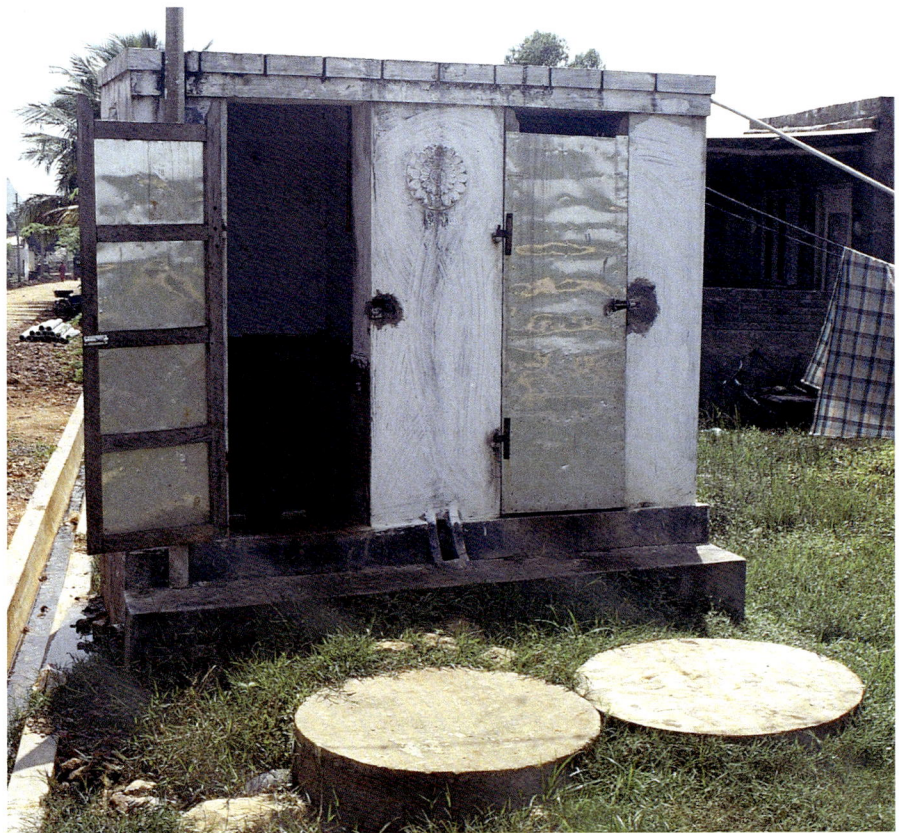

Intercountry and interregional interaction

What happened after the Beppu Declaration?

EASAN1 contributed decisively to promoting the advancement of the difficult agenda of improving the sanitation status in most countries in East Asia. However, it is difficult, if at all attainable, to measure unequivocally the actual contribution of these initiatives to sanitation sector development at the country level.

The activities put into effect or strengthened following EASAN1, reported through the TWG WHS templates, range from national promotion and advocacy events in several East Asian countries to initiatives with exceedingly relevant impact such as the formulation of the Philippine national roadmap on sanitation and the Chinese policy decision to build or upgrade tap water supply systems and a wash room for each family in rural China.

BOX 9 The International Year of Sanitation

Recognition of the sanitation crisis prompted the United Nations to declare 2008 "The International Year of Sanitation (IYS)" and to invite its Member States and organizations and supporters worldwide to get involved. The IYS provides an opportunity to draw attention to the needs of over one-third of global citizens for the most basic services by promoting five key messages concerning sanitation and to generate new resources to address the crisis at international, national and community levels.

Sanitation is vital for health
Lack of toilets and the safe confinement of excreta away from hands, feet, drinking-water and eating utensils and lack of hygiene, especially a failure to wash hands after defecation, lead to the transmission of diarrhoeal disease. Sanitation is important for the prevention of all illness and saves huge medical costs.

Sanitation contributes to social development
Where sanitation facilities and hygienic behaviour are present, rates of illness drop, malnutrition in children is reduced, more children, especially girls, attend school and learn better and women's safety and dignity are enhanced.

Sanitation is a good economic investment
Improved sanitation has positive economic benefits. Livelihoods and employment opportunities are enhanced and the costs of illness and lost productivity to the community and the nation are reduced.

Sanitation helps the environment
Improved disposal of human waste promotes environmental cleanliness and protects streams, rivers, lakes and underground aquifers from pollution. Safely composted, excreta can be used as fertilizer.

Sanitation is achievable
Tried and tested appropriate technologies, programme models and people-centred approaches can be rolled out where there is the will to do so. The cost of meeting the MDG sanitation target is affordable.

Source: UN-Water (2008)

* UN-Water is a mechanism of the United Nations to support states in their water-related efforts to reach the MDG. It was officially endorsed in 2003 as a follow-up to the 2002 World Summit on Sustainable Development.

A crucial resolution of EASAN1 was the creation of a regional platform for cooperation in sanitation and hygiene, which should include an East Asia Ministerial Conference on Sanitation and Hygiene to be organized biennially. This resolution proved to be highly relevant because it allowed the establishment of mechanisms for an exchange of information and follow-up to the resolutions signed by the ministers of state attending this significant event.

What can be done to enhance cooperation and exchange of information among East Asian countries?

The consensus is that the focus should be on regional promotion and advocacy, improving country-level sector monitoring and creating the technical tools and support for national training programmes as summarized in Table 9.

TABLE 9   How to enhance cooperation and exchange of information among East Asian countries

Countries recommending	Recommendation
China	The countries of the Region should play a more active role in the collective regional and global efforts to improve sanitation and hygiene.
Indonesia Mongolia Viet Nam	More frequent meetings of East Asian countries for increased face-to-face exchanges of information.
Brunei Darussalam Cambodia Indonesia The Lao People's Democratic Republic The Philippines The Republic of Korea Viet Nam	Generate training opportunities among the countries of the Region in terms of cross-country study tours, organizing intercountry workshops and other training activities.
Cambodia Indonesia The Lao People's Democratic Republic The Philippines Viet Nam	Establish a joint Internet information system for enhanced networking and exchange of information.
Cambodia China	Disseminate best practice documents and prepare new tools (guidelines, manuals and training packages) to fill information gaps. Establish the mechanisms for information dissemination within the Region (newsletter, listserv).
The Philippines	Joint regional project preparation and implementation.

Source: TWG WHS templates

Way Forward

The MDG sanitation target is unlikely to be reached for East Asia as a whole and for many countries individually. Even if the MDG target is attained, it still means that a half billion people in the Region will have no access to improved sanitation in 2015. Achieving the MDG target will require that the Region double its annual level of investment in sanitation until 2015.

There should be longer-term planning. The East Asian countries would benefit greatly from earlier planning for the years beyond 2015.

There should be a more comprehensive examination of sanitation. The definition of basic sanitation adopted in this document calls for sanitation systems that are sustainable, hygienic, affordable and ensure a healthful environment both at home and in the neighbourhood of users. This entails the need to address crucial issues such as wastewater treatment and disposal in a realistic and effective way. For example, as the proportion of people in urban areas with access to home water supply from centralized piped systems increases steadily, the volume of urban wastewater generated certainly increases at a similar rate. Ignoring such a trend will certainly bring about damaging consequences to the health and economy of people downstream and will harm the environment because of raw wastewater discharged indiscriminately into receiving bodies of water. There should be a requirement to examine on-site sanitation, taking into account the need for health protection, cleanliness, environmental protection, sustainability and affordability. Many on-site sanitation facilities deemed "improved" may be contaminating groundwater sources used for domestic supply.

Measures for achieving an East Asia with adequate and sustainable sanitation for all

The TWG WHS Member States indicated the priorities and required action to advance the sanitation agenda in the Region. This is reflected throughout this document. When requested to summarize the main measures for achieving an East Asia with adequate and sustainable sanitation for all their responses were as follows:

Policies and strategies

- A national policy on sanitation is a crucial need. It must be formulated by the appropriate national institution in close consultation with all concerned stakeholders in the sector. Hygiene promotion should be an integral part of such a policy.
- Issuing a national policy is an important step towards better sanitation and hygiene. There is also a need for continuous promotion, provision of technical and financial support and monitoring of action derived from this policy.
- Country-level sanitation action should be undertaken through a sound national programme, clear definition of targets and a realistic action and investment plan.
- Sanitation policies and programmes should be formulated independently from other priority areas. For example, bundling sanitation with water supply or water resources management might jeopardize the effective implementation of the former.

Legal framework

- Prepare an inventory of existing laws, decrees, regulations and similar instruments and undertake the required action to update them accordingly.
- Build a strong and modern legal and controlling framework (laws, decrees, regulations) based on the reality of the sanitation situation and one that is supportive of creating a better quality universal access to sanitation.
- The legal and regulatory framework for sanitation should recognize different national and subnational requirements and should be formulated by taking such differences into account.

Institutional framework

- While sanitation functions preferably should be decentralized, it is fundamental to have a well-established national lead agency with the institutional mandate to coordinate the sector and provide routine financial and technical support at all levels.
- The functions of the various sanitation stakeholders should be defined clearly to avoid overlapping responsibilities and sector gaps. Where gaps exist, the appropriate institutional measures should be undertaken to bridge such gaps.
- Institute mechanisms for coordination and exchange of information at the national level. A sanitation and hygiene committee at the highest possible level would serve as major support for effective country coordination and collaboration. Where this mechanism already exists, it should be strengthened and have a special focus on sanitation and hygiene.

Financing

- There is definitely a pressing need for increasing the national and subnational budgets for sanitation and establishing better financing arrangements to expedite action at all levels.
- Financial resources dedicated to sanitation should concern all stakeholders -- national and local governments, international organizations, NGOs, bilateral agencies, communities and the users. However, the ultimate responsibility for mobilizing resources (human, financial) for sanitation is at the government level, whether national or subnational.
- Scarce financial resources for sanitation should be used wisely. In addition to seeking increased financial allocations from the government and an increasing external budget from donors, local governments and communities should be encouraged to implement total sanitation campaigns or similar approaches which put people at the centre of concerns and stimulate local public and private entrepreneurship.

Monitoring and evaluation

- A national unified sanitation and water sector monitoring and assessment system should be established under the coordination of a clearly empowered national government agency. Such a system should include recurrent assessments and respective reporting and a database accessible to all stakeholders.
- Increase the financial and human resources for monitoring and evaluation to realistic levels so they can be performed effectively and usefully.
- All stakeholders should be viewed as users of and contributors to monitoring and evaluation of sanitation and hygiene. However, these roles and responsibilities need to be clarified for better efficiency of the system and to avoid conflicting information or information gaps.

Capacity building

- Human resources preparation at all levels, including training, should be a fundamental priority in the sanitation and hygiene sector. However, preparing human resources should be based on a solid strategy, which includes not only training but also recruitment, career advancement, motivation and realistic salaries.
- Although training of sanitation staff is needed at all levels, it is fundamental to have well-trained managers both at the national and local government levels.

- Increase the quantity and quality of human resources dedicated to sanitation and hygiene through a realistic allocation of financial resources and targeted training.

Recommendations for strategic or technical sanitation action at the country level were also well-formulated in the EASAN1 discussion document. Box 10 below summarizes the "Things to do in East Asia," proposed in the foregoing document.

How to organize the EASAN platform?

The considerations below were inspired by the analysis of country-based information from both the TWG WHS sanitation templates and strategic resolutions adopted at EASAN1. Two of these crucial resolutions call for "strengthening regional cooperation between and amongst our countries to facilitate sharing of knowledge to expedite change and to create a regional platform for cooperation in sanitation and hygiene" (WHO, WSP, UNICEF 2008).

The crucial questions are what should be the focus of such interaction and how to facilitate collective action of the Member States to ensure the improvement of sanitation locally. The text below focuses on collaborative frameworks that would generate country-level benefits if handled collectively at the regional level.

The following issues and suggestions are intended to provide discussion points on strengthening and putting into operation the regional platforms for cooperation in sanitation and hygiene. First, the two existing regional sanitation platforms operational in East Asia (EASAN and TWG WHS) basically have similar objectives and most of the Member States have both platforms in common. Mainstreaming these two platforms into one unified Regional arrangement for sanitation might be necessary if a more efficient use of regional resources is to be achieved. For example, the TWG WHS could provide the permanent secretariat to the EASAN platform.

Second, there should be a clear definition of the objectives, scope and mechanisms of a functioning EASAN platform. It focuses currently on organizing biennial ministerial sanitation conferences to provide a forum for regional discussion and regional resolutions in the expectation that such resolutions will be translated into action at the country level. This mechanism so far has been useful in raising awareness and generating commitment at a high policy-making level, but its efficacy might be fading as time elapses. There should be an evolution from regional deliberations and reiteration of support for the sanitation agenda to action of more direct benefit to Member States.

Third, there should be financial support for the EASAN platform from multilateral and bilateral agencies active in the Region. Converting the

---

BOX 10 Things to do in East Asia

1. **Improve the enabling environment – prevent sanitation from being submerged by water supply:** Form a separate sanitation working group and formulate separate sanitation policies.

2. **Conduct a national cost-effectiveness review:** Use a review of the relative cost-effectiveness of different sanitation interventions to build consensus on the methodologies, institutional structures and implementation mechanisms needed for large-scale sanitation improvement.

3. **Use Outcome-Based Incentive Frameworks to drive large-scale sanitation improvement:** Monitor a wider range of sanitation outcomes and create incentive frameworks that reward the achievement of pre-defined sanitation outcomes.

4. **Formulate national sanitation plans and programmes (for universal sanitation):** Formulate a long-term strategic action plan.

Source: WSP, WHO, UNICEF (2007)

EASAN platform from a recurrent regional forum to an organized collective effort towards country action will require additional technical and financial backup beyond what is currently available.

Based on the above considerations, it is suggested that the following issues should be discussed and agreed among EASAN Member States:

Scope of the EASAN platform

According to the perceptions and needs interpreted from the analysis of the TWG WHS templates, the following are issues of greater interest to Member States:

- **Regional forums:** Continue organizing regional forums for exchange of information and ministerial conferences to stimulate sanitation promotion, policy-making and sanitation improvement at the country level.
- **Exchange of information:** Establish suitable mechanisms for exchange of technical and strategic information on sanitation improvement.
- **Sector monitoring and assessment:** Support Member States in establishing sound sanitation sector monitoring and assessment programmes capable of generating reliable information for policy-making, strategic planning and programming.
- **Training:** Create tools, training packages and workshops for training of trainers on sanitation issues of common concern to all Member States.

Organizational framework

Steering Committee

The EASAN's Steering Committee membership should be composed of delegates appointed by the Member States. The frequency, scope and other details of each meeting of the Steering Committee should be defined and agreed within a reasonable time frame.

Secretariat

If EASAN platform evolves from the organization of regional ministerial conferences to also accommodate the needs of the sector with regard to information, tool development, training and information exchange, there would be a need for a secretariat that will plan and organize the activities of EASAN in consultation with the EASAN Steering Committee. Four different scenarios are devised in this document for establishing such a secretariat:

Scenario 1: The EASAN process will be assumed by the TWG WHS secretariat. The latter will organize the overall functions of EASAN platform, with support from international organizations such as WHO, WB/WSP, UNICEF, the Asian Development Bank (ADB), the United Nations Economic and Social Commission for Asia and the Pacific (UNESCAP) and others.

Advantages: The regional framework for sanitation will be streamlined, avoiding duplication and overlapping. It is more effective to have one strong regional initiative than two initiatives dealing with similar issues and relying basically on the same people and same institutions. It will be easier to raise financial support for just one unified regional initiative.

Disadvantages: The TWG WHS secretariat might be overwhelmed with the sanitation activities of EASAN, especially if external funding is inadequate.

Scenario 2: EASAN will establish its own secretariat arrangements. In order to ensure ownership and legitimacy, EASAN's secretariat should be hosted by one of the signatory countries of the Beppu Declaration with support from external agencies where needed.

Advantages: A secretariat entirely devoted to EASAN might function more effectively.

Disadvantages: It might be difficult to find a Member State that will volunteer to host the EASAN secretariat continuously. The multilateral and bilateral agencies supporting both EASAN and the TWG WHS would be overburdened by the extra effort of conveying financial support to two parallel similar initiatives. The activities of EASAN and TWG WHS might overlap.

Scenario 3: EASAN would have a rotating secretariat hosted by one of the Member States to be established at each regional forum.

Advantages: It would allow Member States to share the burden of keeping the EASAN secretariat.

Disadvantages: The EASAN secretariat could prove unstable if not enough Member States would be willing to participate in a rotating schedule. Each change of a host country would mean the involvement of different local supporting staff, which possibly would not be well acquainted with the overall EASAN platform. External funding for a rotating secretariat might be more difficult.

Scenario 4: The scope of the EASAN platform as suggested by the respondents to the TWG WHS template is not feasible. Under this scenario, EASAN will continue operating under the same procedural schedule as now, with the EASAN platform devoted basically to the organization of recurrent regional ministerial conferences with the support of partner international organizations such as WHO, UNICEF, WB/WSP, (UNESCAP), the United Nations Environmental Program (UNEP) and others.

Advantages: The current procedure for organizing the EASAN platform conferences has proved to be effective and future conferences are likely to be organized without difficulty. No fixed secretariat or activities between conferences would be necessary, which would minimize costs.

Disadvantages: The EASAN platform will not respond totally to the aspirations of its membership. The platform will be limited to the biennial regional conferences without structured activities between these events. The impact and attractiveness of these conferences might fade as time passes.

Membership

Theoretically, the Member States should include all 16 East Asian countries, which together have 2.1 billion people (about 30% of the world's population). The signatories of the Beppu Declaration are assumed to be confirmed Member States of the EASAN platform. An effort should be made to add the remaining East Asian countries as official signatories of this international initiative.

Work Plan

In the event any of the initial three scenarios is adopted, a work plan should be prepared containing a clear definition of tasks, responsibilities and financial requirements accordingly. Such a plan should be monitored effectively by the secretariat and updated periodically.

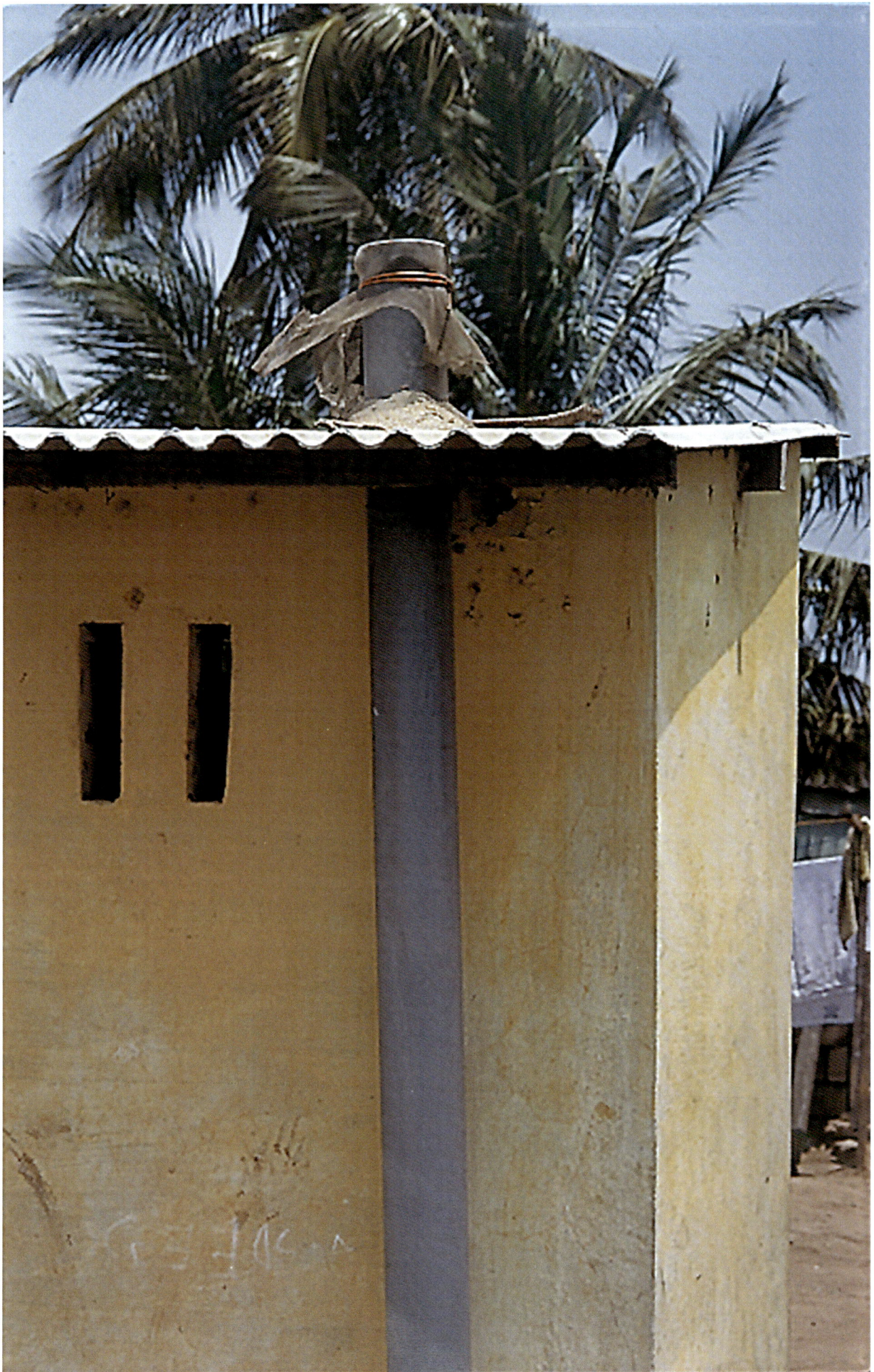

Bibliographic references

ADB et al., 2006. *Asia Water - Are Countries in Asia on track to meet Target 10 of the Millennium Development Goals?*, Manila: Asian Development Bank.

Evans, B., 2004. Whatever happened to sanitation: practical steps to achieving a core development goal. Available at: http://www.irc.nl/docsearch/title/125849 [Accessed November 19, 2009].

Fewtrell et al., 2005. Water, sanitation, and hygiene interventions to reduce diarrhoea in less developed countries: a systematic review and meta-analysis. Lancet Infectious Diseases. *Lancet Infectious Diseases*, 5(1), 42-52.

Hutton G et al., 2008. *Economic impacts of sanitation in Southeast Asia: summary report*, Jakarta: World Bank, Water and Sanitation Program. Available at: http://www.wsp.org/UserFiles/file/Sanitation_Impact_Synthesis_2.pdf [Accessed November 9, 2009].

Hutton, G. & Bartram, J., 2008. *Regional and Global Costs of Attaining the Water Supply and Sanitation Target (Target 10) of the Millennium Development Goals*, Geneva: World Health Organization.

Lenton, R., Wright, A. & Lewis, K., 2005. *Health, dignity and development: what will it take?*, New York: Water and Sanitation Task-force for the Millennium Project.

Mehta, M. & Knapp, A., 2004. The challenge of financing sanitation for meeting the Millennium Development Goals.

Mukalla, R., 2008. Scaling up safe sanitation in South Asia.

Prüss-Üstün A et al., 2008. *Safer water, better health: costs, benefits and sustainability of interventions to protect and promote health*, Geneva: World Health Organization.

UN, World Population Prospects: The 2008 revision population. *United Nations Population Division*. Available at: http://esa.un.org/unpp/index.asp?panel=5#Asia [Accessed December 1, 2009].

UN Water, 2008. Tackling a global crisis – International Year of Sanitation 2008. Available at: http://esa.un.org/iys/docs/IYS_flagship_web_small.pdf [Accessed October 7, 2009].

UNICEF, 2009. Sanitation and hygiene - Case study No. 5. Available at: http://www.unicef.org/wash/files/5_case_study_CAMBODIA_final_web.pdf [Accessed November 5, 2009].

UNICEF & WHO, 2009. *Diarrhoea: Why children are still dying and what can be done*, New York: United Nations Children's Fund.

Wagner, K. & Lanoix, J., 1958. *Excreta Disposal for Rural Areas and Small Communities*, Geneva, Switzerland: World Health Organization.

WHO, 2006. *Guidelines for the safe use of wastewater, excreta and greywater*, Geneva: World Health Organization.

WHO, 2009a. Improving national systems to monitor access to drinking-water and sanitation. Unpublished.

WHO, 1999. *The Evolution of Diarrhoeal and Acute Respiratory Disease Control at WHO*, Geneva, Switzerland: World Health Organization. Available at: http://whqlibdoc.who.int/hq/1999/WHO_CHS_CAH_99.12.pdf [Accessed October 25, 2009].

WHO, 2003. *The world health report 2003*, Geneva, Switzerland: World Health Organization.

WHO, 2009b. *World Health Statistics 2009*, Geneva: World Health Organization.

WHO & DFID, 2009. *Vision 2030 – The resilience of water supply and sanitation in the face of climate change - Summary and policy implications*, Geneva: World Health Organization.

WHO & UNEP, 2007. Charter of the regional forum on environment and health Southeast and East Asian countries - framework for cooperation. In Bangkok, Thailand: WHO Western Pacific Regional Office.

WHO & UNICEF, *Global water supply and sanitation assessment 2000 report*, Geneva: World Health Organization.

WHO, WSP & UNICEF, 2008. Conference report. In Beppu City, Japan, from 30 November to 1 December 2007: WHO Western Pacific sRegional Office, Manila.

WHO & UNICEF, 2008. *Progress on Drinking Water and Sanitation: Special Focus on Sanitation*, New York. Available at: http://www.wssinfo.org/en/40_MDG2008.html [Accessed November 9, 2009].

WHO/WPRO & SOPAC, 2008. *Sanitation, hygiene and drinking-water in the Pacific island countries: Converting commitment into action*, Manila: WHO Western Pacific Regional Office.

WHO/WPRO & UNICEF/EAPRO, 2009. *Establishing a drinking-water and sanitation sector assessment process: a guide for country-level action*, Manila: WHO Western Pacific Regional Office.

WHO/WPRO & UNICEF/EAPRO, 2008. *Water supply and sanitation sector assessments: a guide for country-level action*, Manila: WHO Western Pacific Regional Office.

WSP, WHO/WPRO & UNICEF/EAPRO, 2007. Universal sanitation in East Asia: mission possible?

Acronyms

ADB	Asian Development Bank
AusAID	Australian Agency for International Development
CBTS	Community-Based Total Sanitation
CLTS	Community-Led Total Sanitation
DANIDA	Danish International Development Agency
DFID	United Kingdom Department for International Development
DGIS	Netherlands Directorate-General of Development Cooperation
DHS	Demographic and Health Survey
EASAN1	First East Asia Ministerial Conference on Sanitation and Hygiene
EASAN2	Second East Asia Ministerial Conference on Sanitation and Hygiene
EASAN	East Asia Ministerial Conference on Sanitation and Hygiene Platform
IWS	International Year of Sanitation, 2008
JMP	WHO and UNICEF Joint Monitoring Programme for Water Supply and Sanitation
MDG	Millennium Development Goal
MICS	Multiple Indicator Cluster Survey
TWG WHS	Thematic Working Group on Water, Hygiene and Sanitation
UNEP	United Nations Environmental Program
UNESCAP	United Nations Economic and Social Commission for Asia and the Pacific
UNSGAB	United Nations Secretary General Advisory Board on Water and Sanitation
UNFPA	United Nations Population Fund
UNICEF	United Nations Children's Fund
UNICEF/EAPRO	UNICEF East Asia and Pacific Regional Office
UNPD	United Nations Population Division
US$	American Dollar
USAID	United Nations Agency for International Development
WHO	World Health Organization
WHO/WPRO	WHO Western Pacific Regional Office
WHS	World Health Survey
WSP	World Bank Water and Sanitation Program

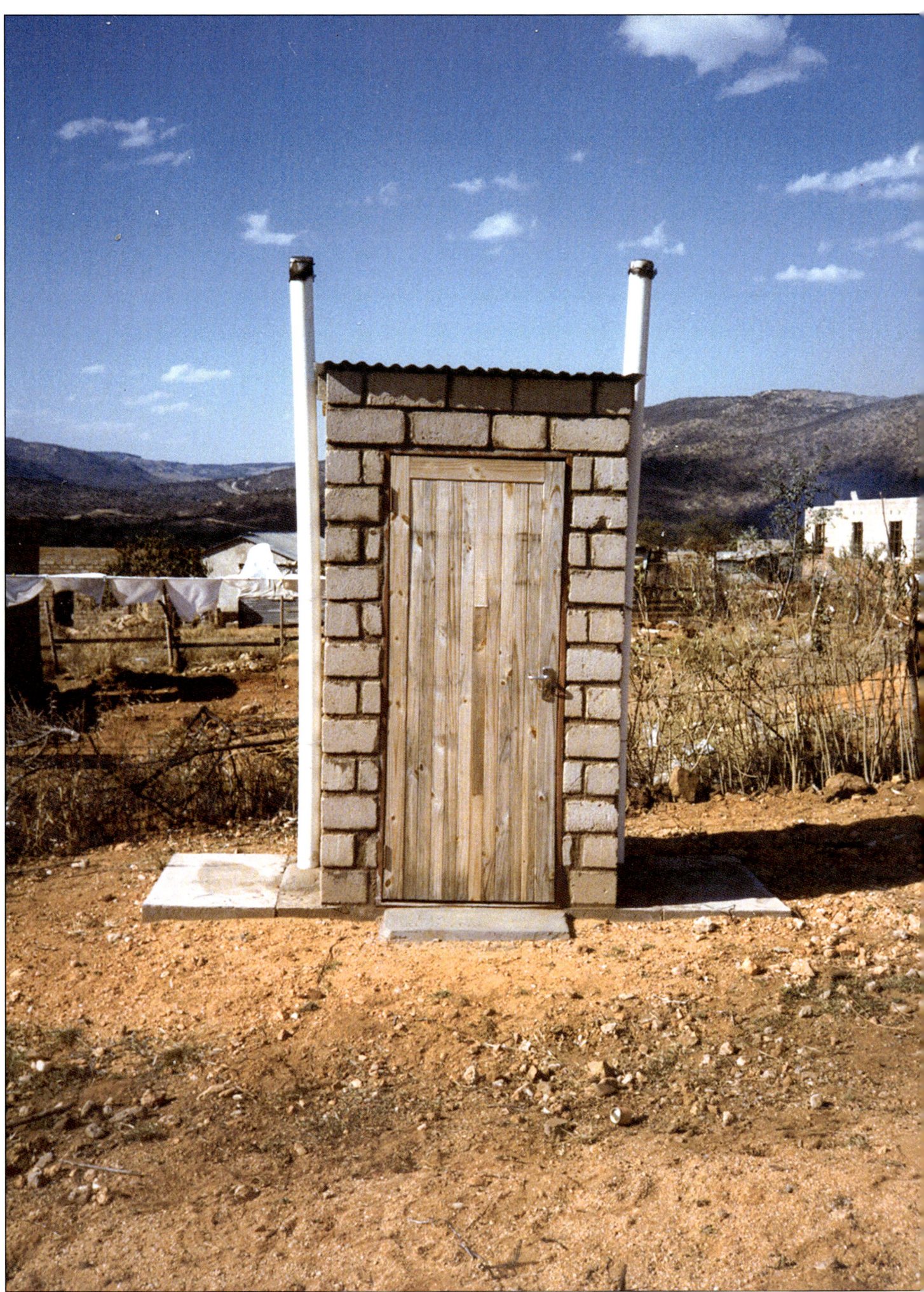

Annex

Annex 1 Declaration of the First East Asia Ministerial Conference on Sanitation and Hygiene

Dated: 1st of December 2007

1. We, the heads of national delegations attending the first East Asia Ministerial Conference on Sanitation and Hygiene (EASAN 2007) held in the city of Beppu on 30th of November and 1st of December in this year 2007 which precedes the UN International Year of Sanitation 2008:

    i. Recognizing that sustainable access to sanitation is one of the targets stated in the Millennium Declaration and that many governments have set their own targets for both sanitation and hygiene
    ii. And further recognizing that sanitation, in combination with the means of practising hygienic behaviours, is fundamental to the achievement of many other Millennium Development Goals which our governments have committed to, defining sanitation as the safe collection, transport, treatment or re-use of human waste along with a healthy living environment including the management of domestic solid waste and sullage, and defining hygiene as clean and healthy behaviours
    iii. And further recognizing that our governments are signatories to the UN General Assembly Resolution number A/RES61/192 which calls for the implementation of the Hashimoto Action Plan including the formation of regional fora to address inter alia the challenges of sanitation and hygiene
    iv. And further recognizing that the governments of East Asian countries approved the Charter of the Regional Forum on Environment and Health in August 2007 in Bangkok, Thailand and the work plans of six regional Thematic Working Groups, including the one on water supply, hygiene and sanitation
    v. Acknowledging that access to basic sanitation and safe water supply and the practice of hygienic behaviours are all necessary for the health and well being of the population and are necessary for people to live in dignity and safety
    vi. Noting that the burden of disease and death and associated economic costs in East Asia which arise from the lack of such access is heavy and is not matched by commensurate investment in sanitation, and hygiene promotion which would, in addition to direct health benefits, have significant economic benefits
    vii. Understanding that national and local governments have a crucial role to play in setting policy and steering public investments to promote a rapid up-scaling of progress in access to sanitation and the means of practising hygienic behaviours while recognising the equally important role of other actors including the private sector and civil society
    viii. And further understanding that the role of households and individuals and particularly women and children are crucial in the realization of effective and sustainable programs for sanitation and hygiene improvement
    ix. And further understanding that effective programs of sanitation and hygiene promotion require the cooperation and coordination of efforts in many ministries including but not limited to those responsible for health, water resources, education and planning

x. And further understanding that there is a growing scarcity of safe water in the region and a linked and urgent need to protect and conserve sources of clean water from both overuse and pollution

xi. Recognizing the depth and value of our mutual experience and knowledge, the availability of positive examples within our region and our potential to act together to improve access to sanitation and the means of practising hygienic behaviours

2. Do hereby commit to

   i. Take the necessary steps in relevant Ministries of our governments at national and local level to achieve or exceed the MDG target for sanitation in our respective countries and to encourage the private sector to take similar steps as appropriate

   ii. Improve the level of investment in sanitation and hygiene promotion in our respective countries while maintaining commensurate investments in domestic water supply

   iii. Invest in sanitation and hygiene promotion in ways which specifically benefit the poor and the vulnerable and those with a high incidence of water- and sanitation-related disease as well as those who currently have the most limited access to sanitation and the means of practising hygienic behaviours

   iv. Plan investments in ways which promote incremental improvements in all needy areas including in the rural and urban contexts

   v. Enable the participation of women, children, poor families, civil society as well as the public and private sectors in the planning and implementation of sanitation and hygiene programs so that they can be scaled to be effective and sustainable

   vi. Strive to ensure that access to sanitation facilities and the means of practising hygienic behaviours are available in all schools and that sanitation and hygiene are a focus of education in schools and that children communicate those messages into the wider community

   vii. Provide strong leadership through Ministries and local governments responsible for finance and planning so that budgetary priorities are linked to workable practical action plans with clear lines of responsibility between and amongst the various concerned Ministries and local governments

   viii. Strengthen regional cooperation between and amongst our countries to facilitate sharing of knowledge to expedite change

   ix. Create a regional platform for cooperation in sanitation and hygiene which would include an East Asia Ministerial Conference on Sanitation and Hygiene to be held in the region provisionally at two-yearly intervals and would build on existing fora and which would facilitate cooperation among East Asian countries as well as between our region and other regions of the world

   x. Play an active role in all the relevant activities and aspects of the International Year of Sanitation.

3. We further call on

   i. Development banks, donors and other governments to support our efforts and provide financial and technical assistance for sanitation and hygiene promotion in East Asia at a level that is commensurate with the challenges ahead

   ii. The Asia Pacific Water Forum (APWF), to recognize EASAN 2007 and its follow-up as an integral part of the APWF process, to recognize this Declaration and to provide practical support in operationalising these commitments

   iii. The G8 and other intergovernmental groups to recognize the importance of sanitation, hygiene and water for global health, for their close interaction with climate change and for the economic and social benefits that they bring

   iv. Other regional fora including the Regional Forum on Environment and Health and the South East Asia Water Forum to also recognize and support this Declaration and assist in converting these commitments into actions

v. Regional and national actors to make use of the opportunities provided by the UN International Year of Sanitation 2008 to maintain and improve efforts in sanitation and hygiene
vi. Relevant Ministries to take strong leadership and to create the necessary environment for effective national sanitation and hygiene programs.
vii. And in recognition of this we make this declaration on the 1st of December, 2007.

Haji Brahim Bin Haji Ismail
Permanent Secretary Administration and Finance, Brunei Darussalam

Lu Lay Sreng
Deputy Prime Minister and Minister of Rural Development, Cambodia

Bai Huqun
Vice Director General, Ministry of Health, P.R. China

Wan Alkadri
Director for Environmental Health, Ministry of Health, Indonesia

Ponmek Dalaloy
Minister, Ministry of Health, Lao PDR

Lim Keng Yaik
Minister, Ministry of Energy, Water and Communications, Malaysia

Shagdar Sonomdagva
Adviser to the Minister, Ministry of Construction and Urban Development, Mongolia

San Shway Wynn
Deputy Director General, Department of Health, Myanmar

Belma Cabilao
Member, House of Representatives, Philippines

Wah Yuen Long
Director, Public Utilities Board, Singapore

Narongsakdi Aungkasuvapala
Director General, Department of Health, Thailand

Madalena Soares
Vice Minister, Ministry of Health, Timor Leste

Nguyen Bich Dat
Vice Minister, Ministry of Planning and Investment, Vietnam

Observers:

UNICEF
UNSGAB
Water and Sanitation Program, the World Bank
World Health Organization

Annex II Charter of the Regional Forum on Environment and Health – Framework for Cooperation

PREAMBLE

Considering the global framework for action provided by Agenda 21 of 1992 United Nations Conference on Environment and Development, the Johannesburg Plan of Implementation of 2002

World Summit on Sustainable Development and Millennium Development Goals of the United Nations, and the recommendations of the 5th Ministerial Conference on Environment and Development in Asia and the Pacific, held in Seoul, Republic of Korea, March 2005 on Enhancing the Environmental Sustainability of Economic Growth,

Recognizing that the environment in which we live greatly affects our health,

Acknowledging the importance of ensuring the protection of human health and the environment,

Understanding that children, the elderly and the poor are among the most vulnerable to and suffer most from environmental deterioration,

Conscious that improving environmental health and ensuring sustainable economic growth are key components of poverty reduction,

Realizing that the maintenance of health and well-being depend on environmental quality and sustainable development;

Underlining the importance and cost-effectiveness of giving priority to preventive action,

Conscious of the urgency to take immediate coordinated action involving all relevant government agencies, organizations from the private sector, civil society, academia and media,

Aware that solutions require inter-disciplinary and cross-sectoral interventions with experts from physical and natural sciences, health and social sciences, development, finance and other fields,

Realizing the specific characteristics, cultural diversity and needs of the region, notably its unprecedented economic development, rapid urbanization and population growth and widespread poverty,

Admitting that nations in the region are physically interconnected by shared bodies of water and air,

Mindful that many environmental and health issues are transboundary in nature and that globalization has highlighted the interdependence of nations, communities and individuals,

Keeping in mind existing international agreements on the protection of the ozone layer, climate change, biodiversity conservation, the management of chemicals and wastes and other initiatives related to environment and health,

Mindful of the precautionary approach and guided by the polluter pays principle and the norms of good governance including civic engagement and participation, efficiency, equity, transparency and accountability,

Taking note of the various efforts being undertaken by various countries at the national and regional levels,

The Ministers responsible for the Environment and Health of the Southeast Asian countries of Brunei Darussalam, Cambodia, Indonesia, Lao People's Democratic Republic, Malaysia, Myanmar, Philippines, Singapore, Thailand and Viet Nam and the East Asian countries of China, Japan, Mongolia and the Republic of Korea, meeting together for the first time at Bangkok on 9 August 2007, have adopted the attached Charter of the Regional Forum on Environment and Health; have agreed upon the principles, vision, goals and objectives, strategies and structures set forth therein as the basis for their joint commitment to collective and individual country actions and call upon their international partners to support the implementation of this Charter.

I. VISION

Sustainable development encompasses nurturing of the environment, enhancing economic growth and social equity to reduce poverty, promoting the health and well-being of people and encouraging partnerships and cooperation among various stakeholders and countries in the region.

We recognize that without environmental and health protection development will be undermined.

Without economic growth, which is essential to poverty reduction and improving the quality of life, protection of the environment and the promotion of health will also fail.

Thus, our vision is to safeguard and enhance health and the environment, thereby promoting the development that reduces poverty.

For that to be possible, the interplay of health and environment and their role in poverty reduction needs to be understood and addressed.

We believe this will be achieved by a national approach that integrates the efforts of various stakeholders in preserving the environment with the protection of human health and well-being.

We also believe that national efforts for environmental preservation and health protection may be affected by development activities and the environmental and health conditions in neighbouring countries. Thus, greater regional partnership and cooperation are needed to address common interests and threats to the region.

II. GOALS AND OBJECTIVES

The general objective of this regional initiative is to effectively deal with the environmental health problems within countries and among themselves by increasing the capacity of East Asian countries on environmental health management.

It aims to strengthen the cooperation of the ministries responsible for environment and health within the countries and across the region by providing a mechanism for sharing knowledge and experiences, improving policy and regulatory frameworks at the national and regional level, and promoting the implementation of integrated environmental health strategies and regulations.

Specifically, this initiative aims to assist countries to:

(1) effectively and efficiently achieve their targets on Health, Environmental Sustainability, Poverty, and Global Partnership for Development under the United Nation's Millennium Development Goals (MDG);
(2) institutionalize the integrated management of environmental health at all levels within each participating country and among the East Asian countries through the setting up of a coordinative institutional mechanism; and
(3) enable countries to assess priority environmental health risks, develop and implement cost-effective National Environmental Health Action Plans (NEHAP) and disseminate the same to the various stakeholders.

III. PRIORITIES FOR 2007–2010

Governments should address the health impacts and implications of the following priority areas of environmental concern at the local, national, regional and global levels:

- Air quality
- Water supply, hygiene and sanitation
- Solid and hazardous waste
- Toxic chemicals and hazardous substances
- Climate change, ozone depletion and ecosystem changes
- Contingency planning, preparedness and response in environmental health emergencies

In addressing these priorities, countries can be guided by the following criteria:

- areas where environmental conditions create or tend to create the greatest burden on disease and mortality;
- emerging significant risks where impact information may not yet be fully available;
- vulnerable population groups; and

- environmental management systems under the threat of deterioration due to aging and environmental degradation.

The importance of multisectoral planning and community mobilization should be kept in mind.

The adoption of healthy lifestyles and other preventive measures should be underscored. The need for joint efforts and regional and international cooperation should be acknowledged.

Capacity building, information dissemination, education, training and further studies should be promoted.

IV. STRUCTURE

The implementation of this Charter will require the formation of an organizational structure to achieve the intent and objectives laid out in this document.

(1) Regional Forum -
 The Ministers of the Environment and Health agencies of the member countries will meet in a Regional Forum which is held within every three years. The Forum shall:

 (a) provide overall guidance to strategic directions and supervision of the initiative;
 (b) ensure the continued quality and relevance of the thematic focus of the initiative;
 (c) formulate recommendations on the implementation of the consensus established by the Forum;
 (d) oversee the implementation of agreements reached during the Regional Forum;
 (e) review activities in terms of consistency with the principles, goals and objectives and priorities defined in this Charter;
 (f) ensure better coordination among member countries and partner agencies in addressing the priorities identified during the Regional Forum; and
 (g) work with existing recognized regional centres as regional collaborating centres for excellence to provide technical support to the Forum.

International partners will be invited to serve as resource persons to the Regional Forum.

(2) Thematic Working Groups –
 Thematic Working Groups (TWG) on specific priority issues will be created. The topics to be tackled will be discussed and approved as regional priorities during the Regional Forum.
 Members of each TWG will come from member countries concerned with a specific issue or have expertise which can be shared to benefit other members. A Chair of each TWG will be selected from government agencies of member countries. Representatives from the private sector, academe, civil society, regional centres, institutions, other regional and global initiatives tackling a particular priority issue may also be invited to become part of the TWG. Attached as Annex A are the terms of reference of the TWG.

(3) Advisory Board –
 An Advisory Board, composed of the Chairs of TWGs and the Chair and Vice Chair of the Regional Forum, will be established. The Advisory Board will meet regularly to review independently scientific information and ensure better coordination among the TWGs in addressing the priorities identified by the Regional Forum and to cooperate with the secretariat in fulfilling its responsibilities in preparing for the next Regional Forum.

(4) Secretariat -
 The WHO and UNEP will serve as the joint Secretariat to support the operations of the Regional Forum and the TWGs. The Secretariat will provide day-to-day management of this regional initiative and will be responsible for:
 (a) collecting information from member countries on significant and/or innovative initiatives related to environmental health management within Asia or where relevant outside the Region, which will include documenting the information in an easily retrievable manner and disseminating it to members through electronic updates;
 (b) maintaining an overview and monitoring the implementation of NEHAPs or equivalent plans developed by member countries to facilitate exchange of experiences among its members during

the formulation and implementation of such Action Plans;
(c) providing technical and administrative support to members who are organizing events that take place under the umbrella of the initiative; and
(d) assisting the Regional Forum in resource mobilization for implementing and expanding activities of its member countries.

V. ENTITLEMENTS AND RESPONSIBILITIES

Every individual is entitled to an environment that permits the achievement of the highest possible quality of life and access to information and participation in the entire decision-making process.

All parties, be they government, civil society including nongovernmental organizations (NGO), media, individuals, the private sector or partner agencies, are accountable for their actions and should evaluate their activities and implement them in a manner that protects people's health and the health of ecosystems. They should actively share information and contribute their resources to the protection of the environment and health at the local, national, regional and global level.

All government agencies, both national and local, should provide a policy that proactively engages others on more effectively addressing environmental health issues. The ministries responsible for health and environment should share information and expertise, make collaborative decisions and work together towards the development and implementation of their NEHAPs or equivalent plans.

It is the duty of government agencies and authorities to protect people in their area and enable them to protect themselves. Authorities are responsible for assessing environmental health risks and environmental management systems within their area and should choose the most cost-effective and affordable interventions to manage those risks and provide the necessary resources to do so. They should also ensure that activities undertaken within their jurisdiction do not damage the environment and be accountable for environment and health of their constituents, other areas, the nation, the region and the world.

The private sector is responsible for assessing the risks commercial ventures impose on the environment and people's health and for adopting measures to minimize them by prioritizing sound preventive strategies, implementing pollution control and investing in research to develop cleaner technologies. They are accountable and liable for any adverse consequences of their operations and products and should integrate corporate social responsibility into their operations.

The media plays a key role in creating awareness about environmental health problems and their solutions, developing values and a constructive outlook that fosters public vigilance towards environmental preservation and health protection. If the media are given access to newsworthy, detailed and accurate information, they can communicate such issues to the general public in a timely and responsible manner.

Civil society, including nongovernmental organizations, plays a critical role in disseminating information, raising public awareness, implementing projects and brokering partnerships which encourage communities, governments and the private sector to work together towards environment and health protection.

Countries and partner agencies of this regional initiative are entitled to access available information on environmental health and are, in turn, encouraged to share information and expertise with the other members.

VI. STRATEGIES

To protect health and the environment a comprehensive range of strategies need to be adopted.

Policies which protect and enhance the environment to improve the living conditions and quality of life of the people need to be put in place through enforceable legislation and other legal instruments. Standards should be based on the best available scientific information and be regularly reviewed to account for new knowledge and emerging technologies.

To address the transboundary nature of some environmental and health issues and to minimize the dumping and transferring of environmentally damaging technologies and products from one country to another, the harmonization of standards and policies should be explored.

Priority should be given to preventive rather than curative approaches through the promotion of healthy behavior and cleaner, appropriate and cost-effective technologies, the adoption of environmental management systems and the promotion of sustainable production and consumption. In this regard, the importance of proper operation and maintenance of existing facilities, plants, equipment and devices should be recognized.

Public–private sector partnerships, such as investment in the provision of essential infrastructure, should be promoted to build on the strengths of each sector to more effectively deal with environmental health issues.

Environment-friendly technologies and products should be promoted while reduction, reuse and recycling of waste materials should be encouraged.

The importance of a healthy lifestyle and personal hygiene should be promoted through effective risk communication, education and other interventions.

Risks and impacts on health should be made together with the environmental impact assessment system.

More studies showing the links between the environment and health should be undertaken at both the national and regional levels as basis for policy and action.

Regulatory tools should be complemented with the use of economic instruments and social networks. User fees, pollution charges and other market-based instruments should be adopted to provide an economic incentive for reducing pollution and risks to public health. The community's social capital and corporate social responsibility should be used where appropriate to enhance their voluntary contributions to the improvement of health and the environment.

More work should be done on the economic valuation of the adverse impacts of environmental degradation on health as well as the benefits of the preventative and corrective actions undertaken to give decision-makers and the public a better understanding of the real costs of damaging the environment.

Public disclosure of environmental performance pressures polluters to comply and governments to enforce existing laws and regulations while recognizing good performers and encouraging them to do better is a strategy which should be more widely explored.

Existing information systems should be strengthened and output made more accessible and shared among countries. For this, an effective monitoring and evaluation system should be set up that provides information on such matters as environmental quality, health impacts, standards and the effectiveness of policies and measures adopted. The evaluation of strategies should be based on relevant indices and if necessary, revised based on the evaluation.

Recognizing that successful and effective environmental health management requires the involvement of a large number of government departments, organizations from the private sector, civil society, academia, labour and media, all stakeholders should be actively engaged in identifying problems and finding solutions, and in the process, building ownership and commitment.

Capacity building of countries, including the use of lessons learned and best available knowledge, should be pursued.

Special attention should be paid to contingency planning and disaster preparedness and response, with priority given to setting up early warning systems.

Technical cooperation should be promoted at every level to support the implementation of national and international environmental health guidelines, to cope with national and global issues and local concerns.

VII. THE WAY FORWARD

(1) Member countries of the East Asian Region should:
- undertake the best possible actions available to address and eventually reverse the trend of environmental degradation and its negative impact on health to ensure the implementation of global and regional agreements such as the MDGs;
- establish and/or strengthen existing interagency and multisectoral technical working groups and national coordination mechanisms/processes and link them with other countries in the region to facilitate capacity building, the exchange of information, technology, resources and learning;
- prepare and regularly update a NEHAP or equivalent plans and ensure its implementation so that priority environmental health issues in the country are effectively addressed;
- build the capacity of various stakeholders to enable their mobilization in support of the implementation of the NEHAP;
- strengthen collaboration among themselves and other regional and global intergovernmental bodies on transboundary, regional and global environmental health issues, including attendance at the Regional Forum;
- strongly advocate for adequate budgets and resources for the environment and health sectors within their countries;
- ensure that this Charter adopted at this meeting is widely disseminated within each country and across the Region in the languages of the Region.

(2) International partner organizations are encouraged to:
- support this regional initiative by providing appropriate technical and financial assistance, information sharing and expertise;
- support the development and implementation of NEHAP and equivalent plans;
- intensify coordination and cooperation among themselves to build synergies, prevent duplication and optimize the use of resources;
- ensure proper coordination with existing intergovernmental processes.

(3) Countries and partner organizations should work for the widest possible endorsement of this Charter to ensure the attainment of its objectives.

(4) Ministers responsible for the Environment and Health of East Asian countries should meet again within three years to assess both national and regional progress and to agree on specific actions to reduce significant environmental threats to health as swiftly as possible.

ANNEX A

Terms of Reference for the Thematic Working Groups (TWG)

To support the achievement of the objectives of the Regional Forum, the Thematic Working Groups (TWG) shall be responsible for:

1. Knowledge management and technical support
   - facilitate the exchange of information, lessons learned and best practices across countries;
   - provide technical support to members through access to specific experts and facilities.

2. Progress reporting to the Regional Forum
   - agreeing on core environmental health indicators specific to the theme covered by the TWG;
   - documenting current status as baseline to benchmark progress;
   - consolidating/synthesizing environmental health progress and impact at the regional level.

3. Coordination and advocacy
   - advocate actions based on the recommendations of the Regional Forum
   - promote the integration of priority thematic actions into the national environmental health action plans or equivalent plans;
   - provide guidance on how existing activities can contribute to the general goals of national environmental health action plan or equivalent plans and the Regional Forum;
   - promote the coordination of various (issue–specific) national and donor-supported activities within the country and the region;
   - disseminate information on activities being undertaken and their impacts.

4. Resource Mobilization
   - Prioritize activities for which funding and other additional support is required; and
   - In coordination with the secretariat, identify possible sources including partner organizations that could support the implementation of said priority activities.

Annex III Sanitation coverage in East Asia in 1990 and 2008 according to the JMP statistics review of 2010

Country	Urban population (thousands)		Rural population (thousands)		Total sanitation coverage (%)									Urban sanitation coverage (%)									Rural sanitation coverage (%)								
					Improved		Sharing improved		Other unimproved		Open defecation			Improved		Sharing improved		Other unimproved		Open defecation		Improved		Sharing improved		Other unimproved		Open defecation	
	1990	2008	1990	2008	1990	2008	1990	2008	1990	2008	1990	2008		1990	2008	1990	2008	1990	2008	1990	2008	1990	2008	1990	2008	1990	2008	1990	2008
Brunei Darussalam	169	294	88	99																									
Cambodia	1221	3137	8469	11425	9	29	2	5	5	2	84	64		38	67	5	9	9	2	48	22	5	18	1	4	5	3	89	75
China	312933	577039	829157	760372	41	55	11	17	41	24	7	4		48	58	25	30	24	6	3	6	38	52	6	8	47	38	9	2
Democratic People's Rep. of Korea	11760	14915	8383	8903																										
Indonesia	54251	117196	123134	110149	33	52	7	10	21	12	39	26		58	67	8	9	16	8	18	16	22	36	7	11	23	17	48	36
Japan	77725	84585	45466	42708	100	100	0	0	0	0	0	0		100	100	0	0	0	0	0	0	100	100	0	0	0	0	0	0
Lao People's Democratic Republic	649	1915	3557	4290		53		3		6		38			86		5		3		6		38		2		8		52
Malaysia	9014	19038	9089	7977	84	96	4	4	7	0	5	0		88	96	4	4	7	0	1	0	81	95	3	4	0	7	9	1
Mongolia	1264	1508	952	1133	50	50		28		9		13			64		31		2		3		32		24		18		26
Myanmar	10159	16145	30685	33418	81	81		11		7		1			86		10		4		0		79		11		9		1
Philippines	30450	58699	31978	31649	53	76	11	15	15	1	16	8		70	80	14	16	8	0	8	4	46	69	9	14	22	3	23	14
Republic of Korea	31740	39234	11243	8918	100	100	0	0	0	0	0	0		100	100	0	0	0	0	0	0	100	100	0	0	0	0	0	0
Singapore	3016	4615	0	0	99	100	0	0	1	0	0	0		99	100	0	0	1	0	0	0								
Thailand	16675	22397	39998	44989	80	96	4	4	0	0	16	0		93	95	5	5	0	0	2	0	74	96	3	4	0	0	23	0
Timor-Leste	154	299	586	799		50		3		4		43			76		5		0		19		40		2		6		52
Viet Nam	13418	24234	52829	62862	35	75	2	4	21	15	42	6		61	94	3	5	10	1	26	0	29	67	2	4	23	21	46	8
Region	574601	985251	1195613	1129692	48	62	9	14	31	18	12	6		63	69	16	20	16	5	5	6	40	56	6	8	38	29	16	7

WHO Western Pacific Region
PUBLICATION

ISBN-13   978 92 9061 483 8